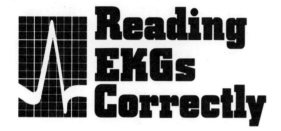

Reading EKGs Correctly

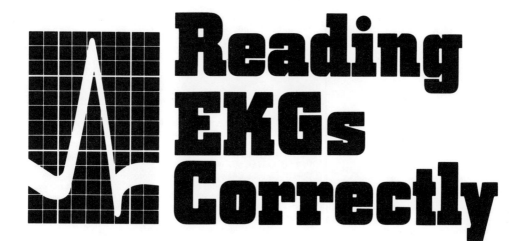

Reading EKGs Correctly

By Margaret Van Meter, RN,
and Peter G. Lavine, MD

Nursing81 Books
Intermed Communications, Inc.
Horsham, Pennsylvania

NURSING81 BOOKS
Publisher: Eugene W. Jackson
Editorial Director: Daniel L. Cheney

NURSING SKILLBOOK® SERIES
Staff for this volume:
Editor: Patricia S. Chaney
Text Editor: Shirley Claypool
Copy Editor: Patricia A. Hamilton
Production Manager: Bernard Haas
Production Assistants: Grace Koontz, Laura Musmanno
Designer: John C. Isely
Art Director: Matie Patterson
Art Assistant: Dale Swensson
Photographer: Bill Baker

Margaret Van Meter, RN, was the clinical director for *Nursing* magazine when this book was prepared. Before joining *Nursing* magazine, Mrs. Van Meter was cardiac care coordinator at Hahnemann Medical College and Hospital in Philadelphia where she was responsible for staff development in the CCU and cardiac surgery ICU. Mrs. Van Meter is a diploma graduate of King's County Hospital School of Nursing, Brooklyn.
Peter G. Lavine, MD, is director of the coronary care division of Crozer-Chester Medical Center, Chester, Pa. Before assuming that position, Dr. Lavine was director of the coronary care unit and assistant professor of medicine at Hahnemann Medical College and Hospital in Philadelphia. A graduate of Hahnemann Medical College, Dr. Lavine is a member of the American College of Chest Physicians. His articles on coronary care have appeared in the *American Journal of Cardiology* and the *American Heart Journal.*

CONTRIBUTOR
Rose Pinneo, RN, MS, contributed much of the material for Chapter 10: "A Glance at Cardiac Monitors." Ms. Pinneo is associate professor of nursing at University of Rochester, N.Y., and clinical specialist in cardiovascular nursing in the Rochester Regional Medical Program.

Library of Congress Cataloging in Publication Data

Van Meter, Margaret.
  Reading EKGs correctly.

  (Nursing79 Skillbook Series)
  "Nursing79 Books."
  Edition for 1975 published under title: How to read an EKG correctly.
  Bibliography: p.
  1. Electrocardiography—Handbooks, manuals, etc. 2. Cardiovascular disease nursing—Handbooks, manuals, etc. I. Lavine, Peter G., joint author. II. Title. [DNLM: 1. Electrocardiography—Programmed tests. 2. Electrocardiography—Nursing texts. WY18 V26H 1975a]
RC683.5.E5V36   1979   616.1'2'0754
ISBN 0-916730-02-6

Contents

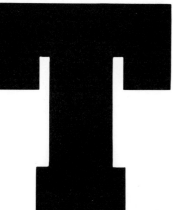

wenty years ago, few nurses knew how to analyze an electrocardiogram. And little wonder; most of them had never even seen one, much less had to evaluate one. Today, though, electrocardiographs, like thermometers, blood pressure cuffs, and stethoscopes, have become standard assessment tools. So, reading and interpreting EKG strips is significant not only for nurses in the cardiac care unit but also in physicians' offices, primary care divisions, emergency departments, and many nursing units in a hospital.

Although the cardiac clinical nurse specialist needs to assess and interpret the more complex strips, the vast number of nurses — from beginners to skilled cardiac nurse practitioners — need a clear, concise understanding of only the most common EKGs. And they want to be able to link this information to their basic knowledge of anatomy, chemistry, and physiology so the rationale behind electrocardiography can be meaningful to them. It is precisely to these goals that the authors of this manual have dedicated their entire approach.

From beginning to end, they have designed explanations to reach the reader at his level of understanding. First, they give a basic account of the electrophysiology and conduction systems. Then, they outline the step-by-step method for analyzing any EKG for rate, rhythm, conduction, configuration, and location of waves. And finally they explain all common arrhythmias, each time focusing on the key questions: Where did it originate? What effect does it have on the heart? What treatment is necessary? What problems might the treatment create? What would happen to the patient if the problem were not corrected? And what are the implied special nursing considerations?

Interspersed throughout are interesting patient studies, so that theory is always linked with practice. At the end of each chapter and at the end of the book, the reader has numerous chances to test what he has learned.

This manual fills a definite need for a compact, interesting presentation of EKGs. By using it, the beginner should gain a rapid but thorough grasp of a sophisticated but relatively simple tool. Then, with continued study and practice, he can build on the basic skills he learns here to become truly proficient at EKG interpretation. With time at a premium, no practicing nurse can afford to pass up this practical manual and the enriching experience of painlessly learning the fundamentals of EKG interpretation.

Lillian S. Brunner, RN, MS, *Nursing Author*
Project Director, Bryn Mawr (Pa.) Hospital School of Nursing

1 What does an EKG tell you about the heart?

Like so much modern electronic gadgetry, the electrocardiograph seems to possess an aura of mystery and magic. Even the terminology of EKG interpretation sounds like an occult code: QRS complexes, inverted P waves, R-R intervals, and so forth.

As mysterious as it all sounds, however, the principles behind electrocardiography and EKG interpretation are fairly simple. In fact, with only a rudimentary understanding of the electrical systems of the heart and the EKG machine, you can make some general observations about a patient's EKG report.

Suppose, for example, you overheard a doctor explaining a patient's EKG as follows: "He's got good P waves and a slightly prolonged P-R interval. But see how much his QRS has widened since last night!"

To generally evaluate the doctor's comments, you need only to know the relationship between EKG waves and cardiac anatomy and to understand which parts of the heart the various EKG leads focus on. More concisely, you

need to know something about the heart's electrophysiology and the 12-lead EKG system.

Electrophysiology of the heart
The many cells of the heart are arranged so that they act as one system or network. Two types of electrical processes, called *depolarization* and *repolarization,* are transmitted throughout this network. During depolarization, the cells are stimulated and the myocardium contracts; during repolarization, it relaxes. The entire process is called the cardiac cycle.

A disturbance in any of the processes of the cardiac cycle will cause a change in the electrical forces needed to maintain normal, rhythmic heartbeats and may produce an arrhythmia. It could be anything from a minor disruption of rhythm to a major death-producing arrhythmia, depending on the degree of the disturbance.

During their resting stage, the cells of the myocardium are said to be *polarized* — that is, they have positive charges on the outside of each cell and an equal number of negative

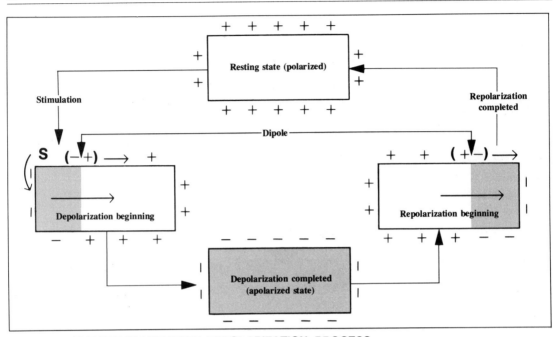

Figure 1 — THE DEPOLARIZATION-REPOLARIZATION PROCESS

charges on the inside. Electrical stimulation makes the cell membrane permeable to the flow of ions, which is responsible for the flow of electrical current throughout the myocardium.

Sodium and potassium ions figure importantly in this electrical activity. In the resting cell, the potassium ion (K+) concentration is 50 times greater inside the cell than outside while sodium ion concentration is greater outside the cell. Upon *depolarization,* the first current flow consists of sodium ions (Na+) moving from outside to inside the cell until the outer surface becomes negatively charged and the membrane is fully depolarized. The flow of potassium ions from inside the cell to the outside begins shortly after the sodium ions start to move in. When the potassium ion flow exceeds that of sodium ions, *repolarization* of the membrane begins, and the outer surface of the membrane again becomes positively charged. This depolarization-repolarization cycle or process is illus-

trated on this page in Figure 1.

This figure also represents a simplified view of the electrical activity of the cardiac muscle. But the architecture of the heart muscle cell and its membrane is very complex. The flow of electrical current through the heart is not simply a transfer of ions across a single membrane; it includes metabolic processes and other molecular activity as well.

To understand the electrical activity of the heart, we must think of the heart as consisting of two separate cell networks — one comprising the atria and the other the ventricles. Stimulation must spread through the muscle of both the atria and the ventricles before mechanical contraction can occur.

Each of these cell networks is considered separately on the electrocardiogram, which is simply a graphic recording of the electrical forces produced by the heart. In fact, all the waves of the EKG can be correlated with the

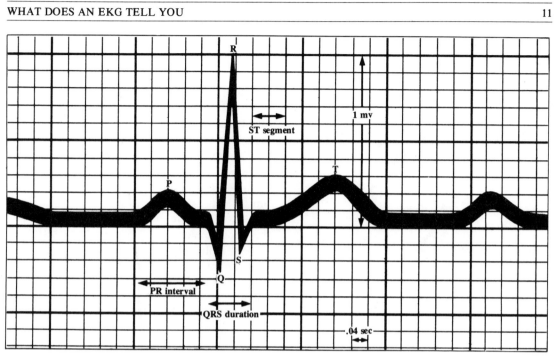

Figure 2 — EKG WAVES FOR ONE CARDIAC CYCLE

level of electrical stimulation that precedes the mechanical contraction and relaxation of the heart. These waves have been arbitrarily labeled the P, QRS, and T waves (see Figure 2).

The P wave reflects depolarization of the atria. The QRS complex reflects the depolarization of the ventricles. The T waves reflect the repolarization of the ventricles. (The T wave corresponding to the repolarization of the atria is not visible, because it is obscured by the QRS deflection.) The mass of the ventricles is much greater than that of the atria, so the QRS and T waves are much larger than the P wave.

Occasionally, another wave will appear after the T wave. Called the U wave, it usually shows up on EKGs of patients who have a low serum potassium. The wave can usually be eliminated by giving a potassium supplement intravenously. (In recent laboratory studies, U waves have been produced in animals during the repolarization stages of the Purkinje fibers.)

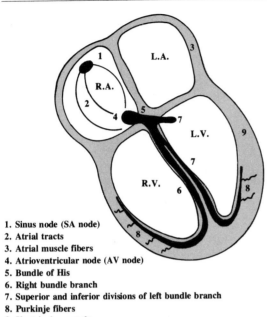

1. Sinus node (SA node)
2. Atrial tracts
3. Atrial muscle fibers
4. Atrioventricular node (AV node)
5. Bundle of His
6. Right bundle branch
7. Superior and inferior divisions of left bundle branch
8. Purkinje fibers
9. Ventricular muscle

Figure 3 — ROUTE OF CARDIAC CONDUCTION

Cardiac conduction

Stimulation of the heart originates in the sympathetic and parasympathetic branches of the autonomic nervous system. The impulse travels first to the sinoatrial node, located in the posterior wall of the right atrium near the orifice of the superior vena cava (see Figure 3). The SA node is the main cardiac pacemaker, from which wave-like impulses are sent through the atria, stimulating first the right and then the left atrium.

As soon as the atria have been stimulated, the impulse slows as it passes through the atrioventricular (AV) node. This node is located near the intraventricular septum in the inferior wall of the right atrium and near the tricuspid valve.

Slowing of the impulse at the AV node allows the ventricles, which are resting (diastole), to fill with blood from the atria. The wave of excitation (stimulation) then spreads to the bundle of His, the left and right bundle branches, and the Purkinje fibers, which terminate in the ventricles. Stimulation of the muscle of the ventricle begins in the intraventricular septum and moves downward, causing ventricular depolarization and contraction. Mechanically, the ventricles empty into the pulmonary (or lesser) circulation and the systemic (or greater) circulation.

The 12-lead EKG system

The basic electrocardiograph has electrodes that are attached to the arms and legs plus a floating electrode for the precordial or chest leads. Most hospitals use a standard 12-lead system that records activity from the frontal and horizontal planes of the body.

The *standard limb leads,* known as leads I, II, and III, are called bipolar leads because each of them has two electrodes that record simultaneously the electrical forces of the heart flowing toward two extremities. That is, lead I re-

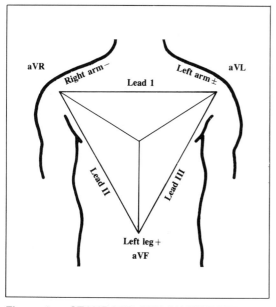

Figure 4 — STANDARD AND AUGMENTED LEADS

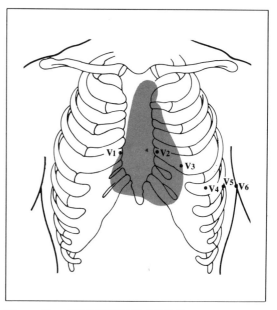

Figure 5 — PRECORDIAL LEADS

cords electrical activity between the right arm and left arm; lead II records activity between the right arm and left leg; and lead III records activity between the left leg and left arm. Figure 4 shows the position of the standard limb leads.

The right arm is always considered to be the negative pole, while the left leg is always the positive pole. The left arm can be either positive or negative, depending on the lead — in lead I, it is positive; in lead III, it is negative.

When current flows toward the positive pole, the deflections of the EKG wave will be upright (positive). When current flows toward the negative pole, the deflections will be inverted (negative). In lead II the flow of the current is from the negative to the positive, so the deflections on the EKG will be upright.

The next three leads are known as *augmented leads,* so-called because they are designed to increase the amplitude of the deflections by 50% over those recorded by the standard limb leads (Figure 4). Augmented

leads are unipolar; they record frontal plane activity, as the limb leads do. Because they record activity from the right and left shoulders and left leg, they are identified as aVR (augmented right), aVL (augmented left), and aVF (augmented foot). By studying all six leads, you will get more information than from the three standard leads alone.

The remaining six leads of the 12-lead system are the unipolar *precordial leads,* or *chest leads.* They are designated by the letter "V" and a number that represents the position of the electrode on the chest wall, or precordium. These positions are: V_1 — fourth intercostal space, right sternal border; V_2 — fourth intercostal space, left sternal border; V_3 midway between V_2 and V_4, on a line joining these two locations; V_4 — fifth interspace in midclavicular line; V_5 — fifth interspace in anterior axillary line; and V_6 — fifth interspace in midaxillary line (Figure 5).

The placement of the precordial leads in rela-

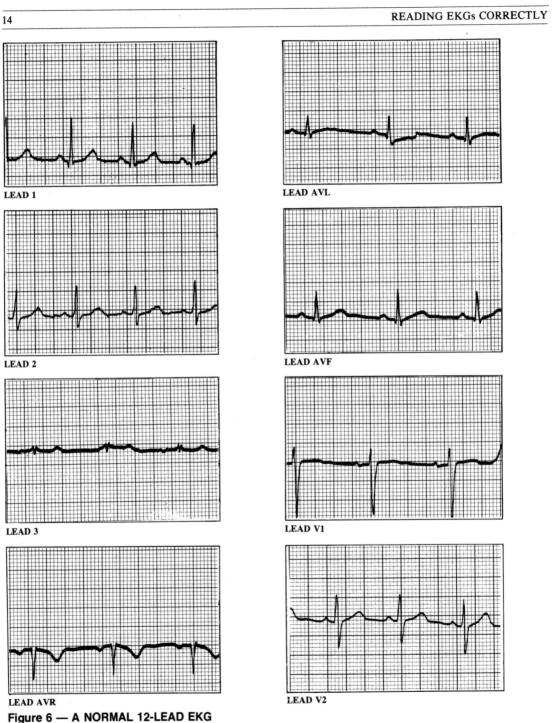

LEAD 1

LEAD AVL

LEAD 2

LEAD AVF

LEAD 3

LEAD V1

LEAD AVR

LEAD V2

Figure 6 — A NORMAL 12-LEAD EKG

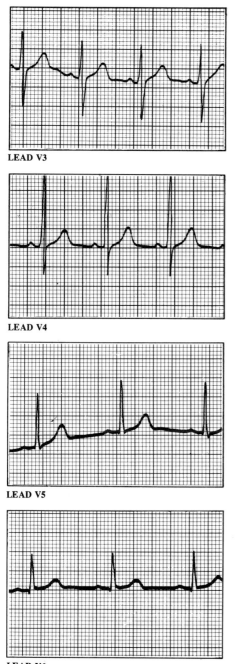

LEAD V3

LEAD V4

LEAD V5

LEAD V6

tion to the ventricles gives a good picture of the electrical activity within the ventricles themselves. Leads V_1 and V_2 represent the right ventricle (and also the right atrium), while leads V_3 through V_6 represent the larger left ventricle. Therefore, these six leads will increase the amplitude of the R wave and decrease the amplitude of the S wave from V_1 to V_6 respectively.

Figure 6 shows normal tracings from each of the 12 leads. If you keep in mind that each lead gives a picture of a different anatomical part of the heart, it will be easy to pinpoint areas of damage or problem areas for the patient.

Applying your knowledge
Now, go back to the doctor's EKG explanation in the beginning of this chapter. With your understanding of electrophysiology and the 12-lead system, can you generally evaluate it?

The doctor's first statement, that the P waves are normal, should tell you that the patient's atria seem to be functioning normally. His second statement, that the P-R interval is slightly prolonged, should lead you to suspect a possible delay in the atrial-ventricular conduction time (AV node). And his statement that the QRS complex is becoming wider should lead you to suspect some cardiac abnormality in the ventricles.

These are educated guesses that you should be able to make from the doctor's general statement. Remember, though, that they are only guesses that you now must prove or disprove. You might discover, for example, that the patient doesn't have a cardiac abnormality in his ventricles at all; instead, the widened QRS was caused by an excess of quinidine. Or you might find that a prolonged P-R interval, if constant, is normal for that patient.

To decide which of these possibilities actually is causing abnormalities in the EKG, you must closely examine the patient's EKG strip, precisely measure the various waves and intervals, and know the patient's history and current treatment. Only then can you determine if the patient has a cardiac problem, where it is, what it is, and what to do about it.

Knowing where a cardiac problem might lie is only a jumping-off point for EKG interpretation; making a thorough evaluation is a much more complex process, which we'll cover in the following chapter as we discuss specific arrhythmias.

THE BASIC EKG COMPLEX: A REVIEW

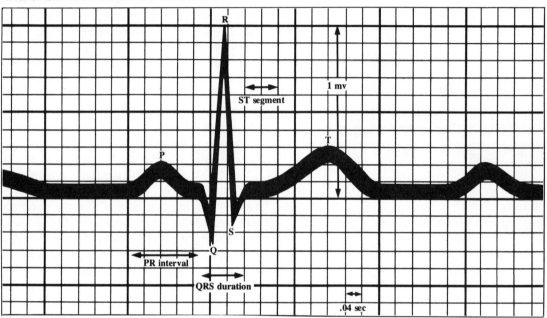

P wave indicates SA node function; produced by atrial depolarization. This wave is best seen in leads II and V1, where it is normally upright.

P-R interval indicates atrioventricular conduction time. The interval is measured from the onset of the P wave to the beginning of the QRS complex.
  - Normal P-R interval: 0.12 to 0.20 seconds.
  - Short P-R interval indicates that the impulse originates in an area other than the SA node.
  - Long P-R interval indicates that the impulse is delayed as it passes through the AV node.

Q wave is the first negative (downward) deflection following the P wave and P-R interval.

R wave is the first positive (upright) deflection after the Q wave. (If no Q waves are visible, the R wave is the first upright deflection after the P-R interval.)

S wave is the first negative deflection following the R wave.

S-T segment is an isoelectric (flat) line having no voltage, from the end of the S wave to the beginning of the T wave.

T wave indicates repolarization of the ventricles; follows the S wave and S-T segment.

QRS duration indicates the time in which ventricular depolarization occurs. Normal duration: 0.06 to 0.10 seconds.

2 Forging a format for interpretation

Imagine you're the night charge nurse on a medical-surgical ward of a 200-bed hospital. It's shortly after 4 a.m. when you get a call from the E.R. that a patient is being admitted to your floor.

The patient, you're told, has suffered an apparent myocardial infarction, but because the CCU has no beds available, he'll spend the rest of the night on your floor. He has typical symptoms: severe, crushing chest pains radiating down his left arm — pain that has persisted despite morphine administered by his family physician before admission. His pulse is 44 and regular (sinus bradycardia); his blood pressure, 90/70. His skin feels cold and clammy; he's perspiring profusely.

On admission the doctor administers oxygen, starts an I. V. of 5% glucose in water, and gives atropine, 0.5 mg I.V. He also orders lab studies: arterial blood gases, electrolytes, cardiac enzymes, CBC, and prothrombin time. A portable cardiac monitor is brought to the floor for continuous monitoring.

Once the physician has left the floor, you check his orders: "Monitor continuously. Notify me of any changes in rate, rhythm, conduction, or of any signs of myocardial irritability such as PVCs, or signs of reduced cardiac output or congestive heart failure. Give atropine, 0.5 mg I.V., for a rate of 50 or below."

Do you know what the physician hoped to achieve by administering atropine, and how to use the monitor to assess the drug effect? How confident do you feel about your ability to pick up changes in your patient's cardiac rhythm? What signs would alert you to deteriorating cardiac output or congestive heart failure?

To answer these questions and others, you first need to know something about EKG interpretation.

Let's begin with a very basic, step-by-step analysis of your infarction patient's rhythm strip (shown in Figure 1) as a practical way of presenting the basic format you can apply to reading any strip. (Although there are other methods you can use to interpret a rhythm

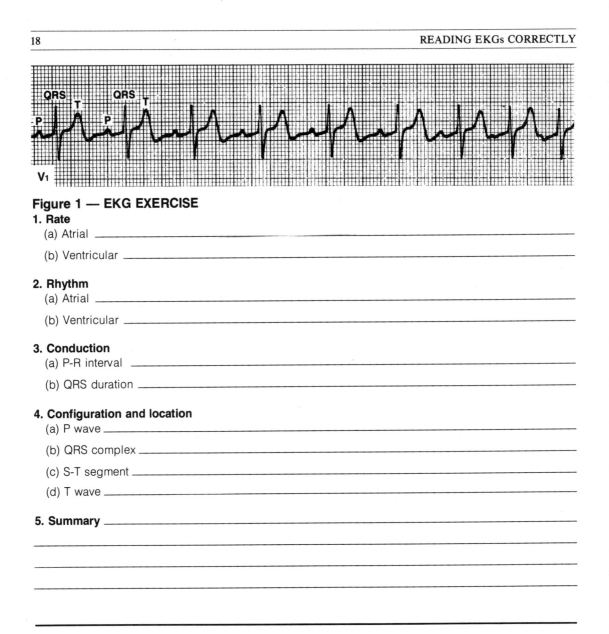

Figure 1 — EKG EXERCISE

1. Rate
(a) Atrial _____

(b) Ventricular _____

2. Rhythm
(a) Atrial _____

(b) Ventricular _____

3. Conduction
(a) P-R interval _____

(b) QRS duration _____

4. Configuration and location
(a) P wave _____

(b) QRS complex _____

(c) S-T segment _____

(d) T wave _____

5. Summary _____
_____
_____
_____

strip, we've found the following method to be the easiest to use.) Unless you routinely work with EKGs, you will probably find working through this analysis a most instructive exercise. Even if you work with EKGs daily in an ICU or CCU, you will likely enjoy reviewing the analysis procedure; however, you will, no doubt, find more of interest in the forthcoming chapters, covering such subjects as atrial and junctional arrhythmias and AV block.

To answer the first question we posed, the physician gave atropine to speed the patient's sinus rate and, in turn, improve his cardiac output and coronary perfusion. By 6:30 a.m., when the EKG (Figure 1) was taken, the atropine had produced the intended effect: the patient's pulse was sustained above 50. The improvement in the patient's heart action was apparent from the EKG (as we shall see); of course, it was also apparent clinically. Indeed, if the atropine had not been effective — if the patient's cardiac output had not improved — he would have felt lightheaded and developed syncope, and even convulsive seizures. If his heart's poor pumping action had persisted, he would have eventually developed signs of congestive heart failure.

Interpreting your patient's EKG
As you read through the following procedure, study your patient's rhythm strip and then write your interpretations in the blank spaces provided beneath it. In this way you'll be developing the information you'll need to report to the doctor when you phone him.

● *Rate.* When we talk about heart rate, we generally mean the ventricular rate, which you can easily feel in a pulse. But to accurately assess an EKG tracing, you'll need to know both the atrial and ventricular rates. First, find the atrial rate.

Since the P wave is indicative of atrial activity, you must first identify the P wave in the rhythm strip (the waves have been labeled for your convenience). Now find two consecutive P waves. Count the number of small squares between the two P waves — you may use either the apex of the wave or the initial upstroke of the wave.

Each small square is equal to .04 seconds; thus, 1,500 small squares equal 1 minute (.04 x 1500 = 60 sec = 1 min). So, you divide 1,500 by the number of squares you counted between the P waves. This will give you the atrial rate — the number of atrial contractions per minute. Write your answer on line 1(a) beneath the rhythm strip.

Now locate the QRS complexes in the rhythm strip. (QRS is more easily identified because it is usually the tallest of the waves on the tracing. Normally, the QRS complex should be 10 small squares high, or 1 mv.) Again, count the number of small squares between the R waves of two consecutive QRS complexes. Divide 1,500 by the number of small squares to find the ventricular rate — the number of ventricular contractions per minute. (If the patient's rhythm is *regular*, you may make your calculations using the calibration table on page 149.) Then write your answer on line 1(B).

(Note: If the rhythm is irregular, counting the squares in a *single* R-R interval will give you an approximate rather than a precise rate, which you would get with a perfectly regular rhythm.)

● *Rhythm.* To determine whether your patient's heart rhythm is regular or irregular, you will again need to know the atrial and ventricular activity. Find the atrial rhythm first, referring back to the two consecutive P waves. For this, you'll need either calipers (see photo 1), or a piece of paper with a straight edge and a pencil with a sharp point.

If you're using the paper-and-pencil method,

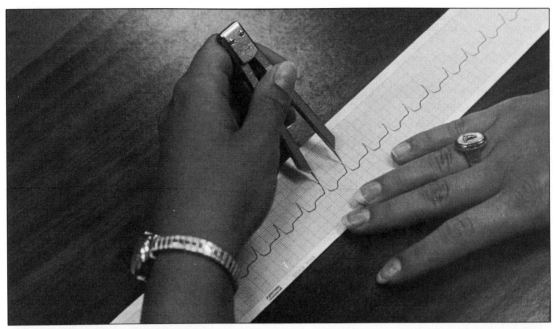

Measure the tracing with calipers

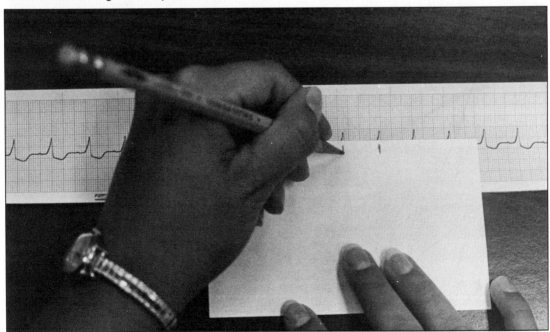

. . . or with a piece of paper

place the straight edge of your paper along the baseline of the rhythm strip. Then, move the paper up slightly so that the straight edge is near the top peak of the P waves. With your pencil, make a dot on the paper at each of two consecutive P waves (see photo 2); this is the P-P interval. Now, move the paper across the strip from left to right, lining up the two dots with each consecutive P wave. If the distance between all of the P waves is the same, the atrial rhythm is regular; if the distance varies, the rhythm is irregular. Write your answer on line 2(a).

Then, using the same method, measure the distance between the R waves of consecutive QRS complexes (the R-R interval) to determine whether the ventricular rhythm is regular or irregular. Record your answer on line 2(b). Note, also, whether the rhythm is only slightly irregular or markedly irregular.

• *Conduction.* Conduction is the time it takes for the impulse originating at the SA node to stimulate ventricular contraction.

Conduction time is found by measuring the P-R interval and the QRS duration. To measure the P-R interval, count the number of small squares from the beginning of the P wave to the beginning of the R wave. Multiply this number by .04 seconds. This tells you how long it has taken the electrical impulse to travel from the SA node through the atria and through the AV node to the bundle of His in the ventricles. Write your answer on line 3(a).

To determine the QRS duration, count the number of small squares from the beginning of the Q wave to the beginning of the S-T segment and multiply by .04 seconds. This tells you how long it takes for the electrical impulse to be conducted through the ventricle. Write this answer on line 3(b).

• *Configuration and location.* The configuration and location of the waves on a rhythm strip also tell you something about the extent and location of myocardial damage.

First, look carefully at all of the P waves. Study their configuration. Are they similar in shape and size? If not, it might mean irritability in the atrial tissue or damage near the SA node. Do all of the P waves point in the same direction — i.e., are all upright, all inverted, or are all diphasic (consisting of both upright and inverted segments)? Is this normal for the lead being recorded?

Next, examine the location of the P waves. Does a P wave precede each QRS complex? Are they present at all? Are they closer to the T wave in some beats? Write your answers on line 4(a).

Next, look at the QRS complexes. Ask yourself the same questions you asked about the P waves: What are their shape, size, and direction; what is their location in relation to the T waves? Also, look at their relation to the P waves.

A QRS complex that is close to the T wave spells danger for the patient because it means that the ventricles, irritated by ectopic stimulation, are contracting prematurely. The closer this ectopic stimulation is to the T wave (which represents the period of ventricular relaxation), the greater the chances of severe ventricular arrhythmia.

Do the QRS complexes occur in groups or clusters — i.e., do two or more QRS complexes appear in rapid succession? Record your findings on line 4(b).

Now look at the S-T segment. Normally, this is a flat (isoelectric) line that is measured from the end of the S wave (of the QRS complex) to the beginning of the T wave. To determine if the S-T segment is elevated or depressed, place the straight edge of the paper along the baseline of the rhythm strip. Look at the S-T segment: Is it on a straight line with the P-R interval? Does it extend above the baseline (i.e., elevated)? Or, is it below the baseline (i.e., depressed)? Record your observations on line 4(c).

S-T segment abnormality provides one of the earliest clues in diagnosing myocardial infarction. (More on this in another chapter.)

Finally, look at the T waves. Evaluate the size and shape of each one in comparison to the other T waves. All T waves should be the same size and shape throughout the tracing. Also, they should point in the same direction as the QRS complexes and should follow them. Record your observations on line 4(d).

In many hospitals, the Q-T interval is also being measured because it gives a better picture of the total ventricular activity. To measure this interval, count the small squares from the beginning of the QRS complex to the end of the T wave, and multiply this number by .04 seconds. The normal interval ranges from 0.32 to 0.42 seconds, depending on the ventricular rate.

Now go back over the findings you've recorded and try to group them so you can report them to the physician. If you find an area in which an irregularity appears, try to figure out whether there is a pattern to the irregularity, or whether it is confined to just one place. For example, if the R-R interval changes with each cycle, you'll know that the ventricular rhythm is grossly irregular. The same is true of the P-P interval.

Now, record your summary on line 5, and compare your answers with those given in Figure 2.

Interpreting your findings
Before your shift ends, the physician calls to check on the patient's condition. You report that he is resting quietly, without apparent pain. Further, the monitor shows his heart rate (ventricular rate) is now 84 beats per minute, with some irregularity in the atrial and ventricular rhythms. The QRS complex has not changed in size, shape, or direction, but some of the P waves have now become inverted. The P-R interval and QRS duration are within normal limits.

The physician interprets your findings like this:

"The presence of P waves and a normal P-R interval preceding the QRS complex, together with a heart rate between 60 and 100 meet the criteria for normal sinus rhythm. (Sinus rhythms are discussed in the next chapter.) You say that when the P wave changed direction, the R-R interval shortened; these irregularities are premature beats, which can be assumed to originate above the ventricles because the QRS did not change.

"Slight elevation of the S-T segment means an irritable area in the ventricles, either ischemia or injury compatible with the admission diagnosis of myocardial infarction.

"Tent-like T waves are often seen with elevated serum potassium, so we'll have to check this electrolyte daily.

"The supraventricular premature beats mean that some atrial irritability is also present. We'll now have to watch the patient for other arrhythmias such as atrial fibrillation, paroxysmal atrial tachycardia, atrial flutter, and possibly junctional tachycardia."

Identifying arrhythmias
What does the doctor's evaluation mean for this particular patient? How can you recognize the various arrhythmias he told you to watch for? As you work through the upcoming chapters, the answers to those questions should become clear. But before we delve into specifics, let's take a look at arrhythmias in general — what they are and what they mean for you and your patient.

Simply stated, an arrhythmia is a disturbance in the cardiac rate or rhythm, or in the conduction of impulses through the heart. Arrhyth-

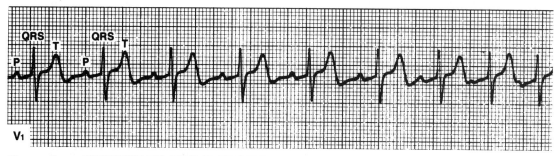

Figure 2 — ANSWERS TO EKG EXERCISE

1. Rate

    (a) Atrial — *84 (1500 ÷ 18) beats per min.*

    (b) Ventricular — *84 beats per min.*

2. Rhythm

    (a) Atrial — *initially regular, then slightly irregular*

    (b) Ventricular — *initially regular, then slightly irregular*

3. Conduction

    (a) P-R interval — *.20 seconds (5x.04)*

    (b) QRS duration — *.10 seconds (2½x.04)*

4. Configuration and location

    (a) P wave — *mostly upright but some inverted; precedes QRS*

    (b) QRS complex — *narrow, uniform size and shape; follows P wave*

    (c) S-T segment — *slightly elevated*

    (d) T wave — *tall, tent-shaped*

5. Summary — *Heart rate is 84 with some irregularity in atrial and ventricular rhythms. The QRS complex has not changed size, shape, or direction. Some P waves have become inverted. The P-R interval and QRS duration are normal.*

The significance of an arrhythmia depends on the patient's cardiac status and systemic reaction to the disturbance.

mias may be caused by several conditions: hypoxia, drug intoxication, electrolyte imbalance, and myocardial damage, to name a few.

The disturbance may be single, such as a rapid heart rate; or it may be multiple, such as rapid atrial rate, conduction delay, and premature ventricular contractions. Combinations of arrhythmias are possible and often do occur.

The significance of each arrhythmia depends on the patient's cardiac status and his systemic reaction to the disturbance. Some patients may be discharged even with a major arrhythmia such as premature ventricular contractions (PVCs); others with relatively minor arrhythmias such as atrial fibrillation may be kept in the ICU.

Whatever the arrhythmia, you'll need to know certain facts to identify and understand it:
1. Where did the arrhythmia originate?
2. What is the heart doing?
3. What treatment would be needed to correct the arrhythmia, and what problems might that treatment create?
4. What would happen to the patient if the arrhythmia were not treated?
5. What special nursing considerations are implied by this arrhythmia?

1. *Where did the arrhythmia originate?* Ideally, all cardiac impulses originate in the SA node, then progress through the atria, the AV node, and the ventricular conduction fibers to the ventricles without any abnormal interference. The presence of P waves on the EKG strip means the impulse did begin above the ventricles.

Hidden or absent P waves mean that the impulse came from the AV node or even the ventricles. In this case, you should examine the QRS complex: Is it wide or normal? A wide QRS suggests the stimulus originated in the ventricles. A 12-lead EKG can best answer these questions, but a lead II or V₁ is a good, quick starting point for assessment.

2. *What is the heart doing?* Is the heart beating too fast (i.e., faster than 100 beats per minute)? Or, is it beating too slowly (slower than 60 beats per minute)? Is the beat irregular? Is it chaotically irregular, or is there some pattern to the irregularity? Is the atrial rate faster or slower than the ventricular rate? If it is faster, can you divide the atrial rate by the ventricular rate to yield a whole number (i.e., 4:1, 3:1, or 2:1)? If you do not get a whole number (i.e., the ratio is not even), something (AV block, for instance) is interfering with impulses passing through the AV node.

Remember, conduction slows somewhat at the AV node and the ventricular conduction bundles, to allow the ventricles to fill with blood, but the delay should be brief (normal P-R interval).

3. *What treatment would be needed to correct the arrhythmia, and what problems might the treatment create?* Until recently, the mainstay of arrhythmia treatment has been antiarrhythmic drugs, notably digitalis, propranolol (Inderal), and quinidine. Although most patients can tolerate aggressive drug therapy, some react unfavorably to certain drugs, presenting obstacles to arrhythmia control. For example, a patient receiving digitalis for atrial fibrillation could develop a more serious arrhythmia (PVC) due to digitalis toxicity.

Other patients will fail to respond to aggressive therapy with digitalis or propranolol and may require a pacemaker or countershock to correct the arrhythmia. However, the presence of high drug levels in his blood increases the chances of cardiac arrest from the countershock.

Nowadays, temporary pacemakers are being used much more frequently to treat arrhythmias because they are both effective and safe if properly positioned, if powered by a good battery, and if supervised by an experienced and knowledgeable nursing and medical staff.

4. *What would happen to the patient if the arrhythmia were not treated?* Sometimes nothing. If cardiac output and tissue perfusion are not impaired, the patient may require no treatment even though the arrhythmia persists.

On the other hand, arrhythmias that impair cardiac output usually must be treated. Rates that are too fast, rates that are too slow, or very irregular rhythms greatly reduce cardiac output. If the left ventricle fails to contract forcefully, blood backs up into the atria and, subsequently, into the pulmonary vasculature. The end result will be congestive heart failure.

An arrhythmia can also create other problems. Diminished cardiac output means diminished perfusion of the brain, kidneys, liver, and myocardium, which in turn causes changes in sensorium and patient behavior, an enlarged and tender liver, and even jaundiced skin. Eventually, the kidney shuts down as the body attempts to conserve its sodium-water balance; the lungs become unable to handle the gas exchanges at the alveolar levels because of the excess fluid backup; and tissue hypoxia from poor coronary circulation to the myocardium will cause the patient to develop more serious arrhythmias besides his original one.

The arrhythmias most important to the patient are those that cause poor perfusion. They are considered dangerous and always require some type of treatment. Sometimes they can be reversed, sometimes not. Whether or not they respond to treatment depends on the condition of the heart muscle, especially the left ventricle. If there is extensive muscle damage, the prognosis is usually very poor.

5. *What special nursing considerations are implied?* You should carefully observe both the patient and his monitor. Even if you're inexperienced in arrhythmia identification, you can notice whether the rate or rhythm changes. You can and certainly should always evaluate

your patient clinically. How does he look? This is your most important clue to his condition. Especially observe his color, behavior, vital signs, and fluid intake and output. Finally, always keep in mind your basic responsibilities: try to give him a feeling of confidence in you and your judgment, try to anticipate his needs, and know when to call the doctor and what he might ask for when he treats the patient.

Systematic practice

With these basic facts in mind, you can begin interpreting the EKG strips in the following chapters. As you do, always keep in mind that the key to learning to interpret a rhythm strip is to keep to *one* fact-finding format. Do not omit any steps. Know *what* you are looking for and *why* you are looking for it. And practice the technique with the strips provided in this book and those recorded in your hospital. If you can find someone to practice with — preferably another nurse — so much the better.

Until you're sure of yourself, write down all of your findings. Then go back and interpret each one as it relates to the others.

If you work in an area that doesn't have continuous monitoring equipment, you can still practice every day by reading the patients' charts and analyzing the EKGs placed in them. If you have a friendly EKG technician, ask her to save excess strips for you, or to run a rhythm strip on the patients on your floor for you to use. Keep a notebook for yourself with these strips and your interpretations. Then compare how your results match up with the cardiologist's when his interpretation is placed in the chart.

In time, *and with lots of practice* (this is the clue), you might surprise yourself with your accuracy.

SKILLCHECK 2

Before going on to learn specific arrhythmias, review the format you'll be using for all interpretation. Measure the following sample strips for rate, rhythm, and conduction. Also evaluate the configuration and location of the P wave, QRS complex, S-T segment, and T wave.

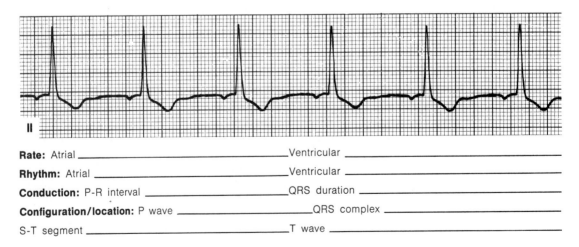

Rate: Atrial _____ Ventricular _____

Rhythm: Atrial _____ Ventricular _____

Conduction: P-R interval _____ QRS duration _____

Configuration/location: P wave _____ QRS complex _____

S-T segment _____ T wave _____

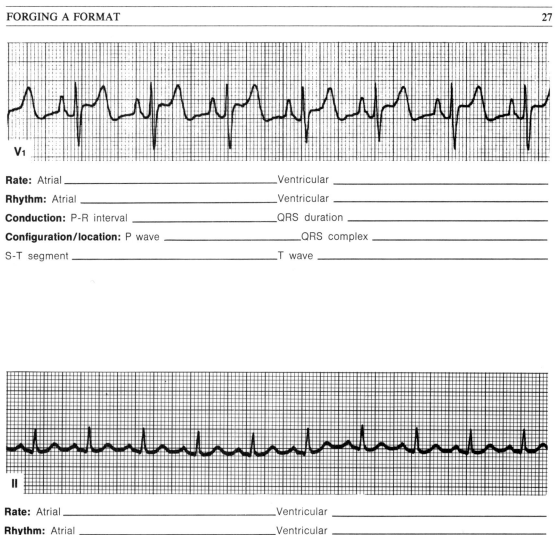

Rate: Atrial _____ Ventricular _____

Rhythm: Atrial _____ Ventricular _____

Conduction: P-R interval _____ QRS duration _____

Configuration/location: P wave _____ QRS complex _____

S-T segment _____ T wave _____

Rate: Atrial _____ Ventricular _____

Rhythm: Atrial _____ Ventricular _____

Conduction: P-R interval _____ QRS duration _____

Configuration/location: P wave _____ QRS complex _____

S-T segment _____ T wave _____

(See Chapter 12 for answers)

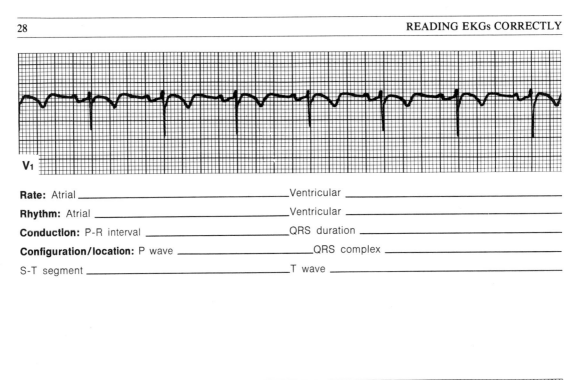

Rate: Atrial _____ Ventricular _____

Rhythm: Atrial _____ Ventricular _____

Conduction: P-R interval _____ QRS duration _____

Configuration/location: P wave _____ QRS complex _____

S-T segment _____ T wave _____

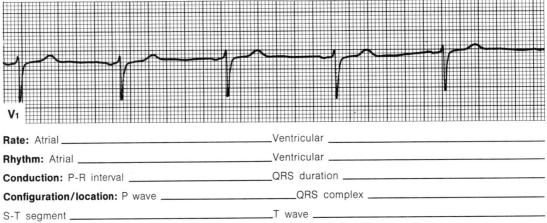

Rate: Atrial _____ Ventricular _____

Rhythm: Atrial _____ Ventricular _____

Conduction: P-R interval _____ QRS duration _____

Configuration/location: P wave _____ QRS complex _____

S-T segment _____ T wave _____

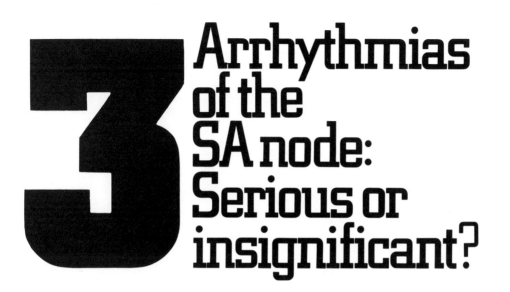

3 Arrhythmias of the SA node: Serious or insignificant?

A good place to begin any discussion of specific arrhythmias is with the most common — those of the SA node. These are generally considered the least dangerous of all arrhythmias. For that reason, many nurses hold the mistaken idea that they are never serious. True, in 99 cases out of 100, they may not be. But in that 100th case, they may indeed be serious, even fatal.

Consider, for example, the case of John S., a laborer who had moderate chest pain for several days and was admitted to our CCU for observation and tests. Whenever the nurse glanced at John's EKG, she saw a normal P wave preceding a normal QRS complex, an apparently consistent R-R interval, and an apparently consistent P-P interval. So, she assumed that John had a normal sinus rhythm. She was wrong. Five hours after he was admitted, John slipped into an atrial tachycardia and from there into congestive heart failure. What had gone wrong? In her casual glances at the monitor and without analyzing a strip, the nurse had failed to detect the minute variations

in the P-P intervals, which indicate sinus arrhythmia and can precede dangerous atrial arrhythmias.

Fortunately John survived. But his experience illustrates just how serious arrhythmias of the SA node can be. It also underlines the first important lesson about EKG interpretation: *You must never take anything for granted.* Just because a patient's EKG appears normal, as John's did, you can't assume that it is without a detailed analysis. Just because arrhythmias of the SA node are common, you can't assume that they are inconsequential. And just because an EKG is a valuable diagnostic tool, you can't assume that it will give you all the answers about a patient's condition. Only by questioning, analyzing, and critically evaluating EKGs and then coupling those findings with information on the patient's medical history, lab tests, and diagnosis can you use the EKG as a valuable assessment tool.

With that in mind, let's examine those common — but not necessarily inconsequential —

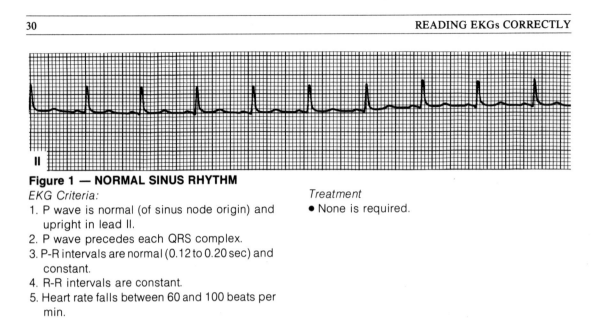

Figure 1 — NORMAL SINUS RHYTHM

EKG Criteria:
1. P wave is normal (of sinus node origin) and upright in lead II.
2. P wave precedes each QRS complex.
3. P-R intervals are normal (0.12 to 0.20 sec) and constant.
4. R-R intervals are constant.
5. Heart rate falls between 60 and 100 beats per min.

Treatment
• None is required.

arrhythmias of the SA node.

Recognizing the norm

Before you can learn to identify any abnormal rhythm, you naturally must learn to recognize the standard against which they are measured — normal sinus rhythm. What is a sinus rhythm? Basically it is a rhythm that originates in the SA node, the heart's pacemaker and the origin of all normal heart beats. Electrocardiographically, sinus rhythms are characterized by the presence of a P wave and a normal P-R interval preceding each QRS complex.

Since the SA node is "programmed" to comfortably initiate 60 to 100 beats per minute, a normal sinus rhythm for an adult falls within that range. But normal sinus rates differ at different ages. At birth, rates of 110 to 150 beats per minute are common. But by age 6, the rates have slowed down to approximately those of adults.

Figure 1 illustrates a normal sinus rhythm. Notice that the heart rate falls between 60 and 100 beats per minute. Also notice the other hallmarks of a normal sinus rhythm: a P wave, always preceding a QRS complex, and constant or fixed P-R, P-P, and R-R intervals. Any deviation from these patterns signifies an arrhythmia. If an arrhythmia originates in the SA node, it will be one of the following.

Sinus bradycardia. In this arrhythmia (Figure 2) the sinus rate is below 60 beats per minute, but all impulses still come from the SA node. Sinus bradycardia may be found in persons whose health is considered normal — especially athletes who have enlarged hearts because of excessive exercise. But it may also be a sign of underlying heart disease, such as myocardial infarction.

Sinus tachycardia. In this arrhythmia (Figure 3) the heart rate is from 100 to 160 beats per minute. Sinus tachycardia may be found in per-

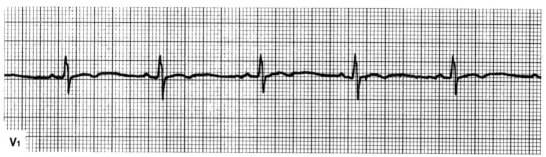

Figure 2 — SINUS BRADYCARDIA

EKG Criterion:
Same as normal sinus rhythm except that the heart rate is slower than 60 beats per minute (thus increasing the risk of PVCs).

Treatment
Patients with signs of poor cardiac output or heart failure may require one or more of the following measures:
- Give atropine, 0.4 mg I.M. or I.V.
- Give I.V. isoproterenol (Isuprel), 0.2-1.0 mg in 250-500 cc 5% glucose in water.
- Insert temporary pacemaker for low output rates, or permanent pacemaker for irreversible symptoms of cardiac damage.

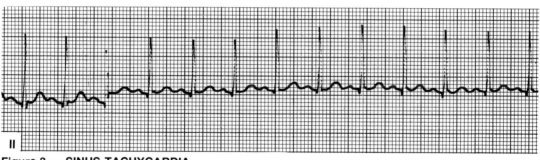

Figure 3 — SINUS TACHYCARDIA

EKG Criteria:
1. Same as normal sinus rhythm except that the heart rate is between 100 and 160 beats per min.
2. P waves are sometimes absent at higher heart rates, but they can usually be found on a 12-lead EKG.

Treatment
- Institute treatment of cause (fever, anxiety, etc.) if it can be determined.
- If heart disease has been diagnosed, watch for signs of congestive heart failure due to fast rate. To treat (or prevent) congestive heart failure, give digitalis and diuretics.

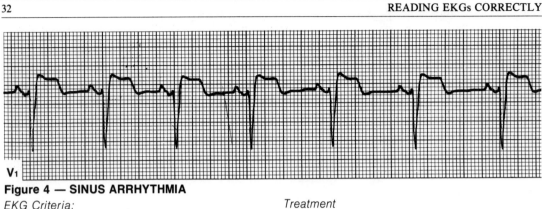

V_1

Figure 4 — SINUS ARRHYTHMIA

EKG Criteria:

1. Same as normal sinus rhythm except P-P intervals vary slightly.
2. P-R intervals vary slightly but within normal limits.
3. Periods of slow and fast heart rates may alternate, especially in children, depending upon crying or respirations.

Treatment

• None is required. However, watch patients with variable P-P intervals for premature atrial contractions and other atrial arrhythmias.

---

sons whose health is normal. It may be related to anxiety or strenuous exercise. Patients who don't have heart disease may experience sinus tachycardia with a fever or with hyperthyroidism. Or, this arrhythmia can be an early manifestation of congestive heart failure.

Rapid rates — more than 160 beats per minute — are considered to originate in an ectopic focus other than the SA node. For many patients whose rate is above 140, P waves will not be visible on the rhythm strip. For these patients, a 12-lead EKG should be taken to determine the exact location of the arrhythmia (atrial, junctional, or ventricular).

Sinus arrhythmia. A normal variation in sinus rhythm, i.e., the rhythm has slight irregularities, is called sinus arrhythmia (Figure 4). Often, a rhythm strip will appear to be normal; only by measuring the P-P intervals all across the strip will you find a slight variation of the atrial rhythm.

The most common type of sinus arrhythmia is found in children and is associated with respiration — the variation of the sinus rate is related to normal inspiration and expiration. That is, it speeds up with inspiration and slows with expiration.

Sinus arrest. Occasionally, the SA node will fail momentarily and will not initiate an impulse. This might be due to increased vagal stimulation (overeating, coffee, cigarettes), pharyngeal irritation (such as that caused by intubation), carotid sinus massage, or deep inspiration (Valsalva's maneuver). This lack of impulse is called sinus arrest, although it is literally an atrial standstill. The atria are not stimulated to contract, so there is no atrial activity.

Sinus arrest may occur in patients who have received excess quantities of digitalis preparation or quinidine. It is not usually of great importance to the patient unless he shows symp-

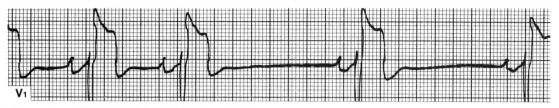

Figure 5 — SINUS ARREST (Atrial Standstill)

EKG Criteria:

1. Same as normal sinus rhythm except that an occasional long pause follows a regular beat (due to SA node failure to initiate impulse).
2. P-P interval is normal except that no P wave is seen during pause in cardiac rhythm.
3. R-R intervals vary because pause is not equal to two regular cycles.

Treatment

- Some patients require no treatment, depending on cause and effect of sinus arrest.
- If sinus arrest is due to cardiac damage near the SA node, insert a temporary pacemaker.
- If SA node is unable to restore normal pacing, a permanent pacemaker may be needed.

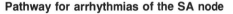

toms of fainting, dizziness, or syncope from the reduced cardiac output.

You can recognize sinus arrest on the EKG by the long pauses, in which beats are dropped. That is, after a normal P wave and QRS complex, there will be no P wave, but rather a pause (straight line—Figure 5). This will be followed by a normal QRS complex. Then the SA node again stimulates the atria.

When this arrhythmia occurs, you should try to determine the cause. Most often, you should watch the patient carefully for the side effects of poor cardiac output. If the patient has organic heart disease from myocardial irritation due to infection or infarction, an atrial pacemaker may be required. This may be either a permanent or temporary pacemaker, depending on prognosis and age.

Wandering pacemaker. An often confusing arrhythmia is the wandering pacemaker, in which the site of the impulse shifts. Sometimes

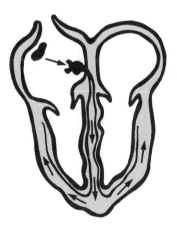

Pathway for arrhythmias of the SA node

Although they're abnormal, all arrhythmias of the SA node still originate in the SA node, which is the heart's normal pacemaker.

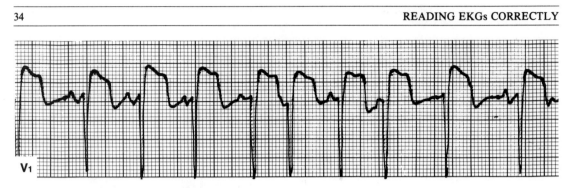

V₁

Figure 6 — WANDERING PACEMAKER

EKG Criteria:
1. P wave changes shape (configuration) and direction because of changing sites of pacing stimulus.
2. P-R interval varies from short to normal.
3. Variations in rhythm occur because of changes in pacing stimulus.

Treatment
- If acute carditis is present, treat underlying infection.
- If due to digitalis excess, hold dosage for short period.
- Observe for other atrial or junctional arrhythmias.

beats originate in the SA node; other times they originate in an irritable atrial focus or even in the AV node.

Because the pacemaker site shifts, the P waves vary in configuration and direction and the P-R intervals vary in length (Figure 6). Ventricular rhythm also varies slightly.

Wandering pacemaker may be caused by inflamed or irritated atrial tissue due to rheumatic carditis or other organic heart disease or by excesses of digitalis. Despite its unusual configuration, it is rarely serious.

SKILLCHECK 3

As you've seen in this chapter, you can differentiate between rhythms of the SA node by checking the heart rate, the configuration of the P waves, and the length of the P-P, P-R, and R-R intervals.

Using those criteria, see if you can identify the following EKGs, which include a normal sinus rhythm as well as some of the arrhythmias we've discussed so far.

Rate: Atrial _____ Ventricular _____

Rhythm: Atrial _____ Ventricular _____

Conduction: P-R interval _____ QRS duration _____

Configuration/location: P wave _____ QRS complex _____

S-T segment _____ T wave _____

Diagnosis: _____

Rate: Atrial _____ Ventricular _____

Rhythm: Atrial _____ Ventricular _____

Conduction: P-R interval _____ QRS duration _____

Configuration/location: P wave _____ QRS complex _____

S-T segment _____ T wave _____

Diagnosis: _____

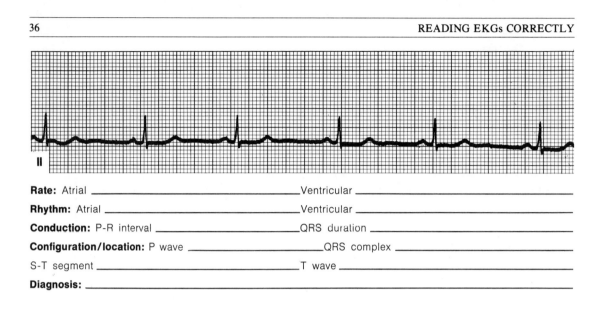

Rate: Atrial _____ Ventricular _____

Rhythm: Atrial _____ Ventricular _____

Conduction: P-R interval _____ QRS duration _____

Configuration/location: P wave _____ QRS complex _____

S-T segment _____ T wave _____

Diagnosis: _____

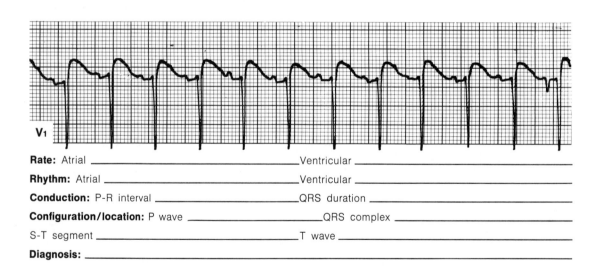

Rate: Atrial _____ Ventricular _____

Rhythm: Atrial _____ Ventricular _____

Conduction: P-R interval _____ QRS duration _____

Configuration/location: P wave _____ QRS complex _____

S-T segment _____ T wave _____

Diagnosis: _____

4 Atrial arrhythmias: Discretion in evaluation

As we noted in the last chapter, it's a mistake to believe that the EKG can supply all the answers about a patient's condition, or even most of them. True, it provides data — valuable data. But only when interpreted in the light of data from clinical observation, laboratory test results, and the patient's history can the EKG serve as a meaningful guide to treatment. This fact was occasionally apparent in our discussion of arrhythmias of the SA node, such as sinus bradycardia. But it will become increasingly apparent in this chapter as we discuss atrial arrhythmias.

A case in point is Dorothy's experience. Her complaint, that her heart was skipping beats, will sound familiar to any of you who have worked the E.R. or CCU. Dorothy was a 44-year-old nurse on our cardiac care staff. Her husband brought her to our E.R. at 2 o'clock one Sunday morning. Both she and her husband were thoroughly frightened, certain that she was having a heart attack.

The E. R. nurse took a brief history while preparing Dorothy for an EKG. Dorothy said she had never had any heart trouble nor could she recall any previous symptoms of cardiac problems before that night. She had been out for a late dinner, had drunk several cocktails and 3 or 4 cups of coffee, and had eaten much more heavily than normal. She had gone to bed about midnight, exhausted but relaxed. At 1:20 a.m. she awoke suddenly, acutely aware that her heartbeat was violently irregular. "It felt," she said, "as if my heart were going to jump right out of my chest. I was afraid that it would stop beating at any moment."

The E.R. nurse first ran a lead II rhythm strip, then checked it while the rest of the 12-lead EKG was being taken. A portion of lead II is shown in Figure 1.

Based on the procedure you learned in Chapter 2, could you analyze the strip? As you work through the procedure, write your findings and then compare them with the criteria for premature atrial contractions (PACs) listed under Figure 2. How do they match?

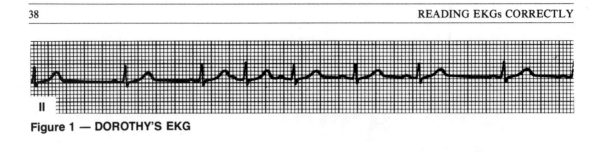

Figure 1 — DOROTHY'S EKG

You should have found that, on Dorothy's rhythm strip, a P wave precedes each QRS complex, although one P wave is almost hidden in the preceding T wave. The P waves differ slightly in configuration. The R-R interval becomes shorter in a few beats, but the QRS complex doesn't change configuration. The two beats following those with the shorter R-R intervals (the PACs) don't occur at the expected time because the SA node — the heart's primary pacemaker — didn't reset itself, or reestablish its timing. Therefore, these could also be considered PACs. Dorothy's diagnosis: normal sinus rhythm with many premature atrial contractions.

How should Dorothy be treated? The clue comes from her history. The premature beats were almost certainly caused by gastric overload plus alcohol and caffeine intake, all of which caused vagal stimulation. (Stimulating the vagus nerve slows the heart rate, leading to the PACs.) So, Dorothy was observed for a few hours and then sent home. She's had no more of these episodes since.

But suppose a patient on your nursing unit complained of skipping heartbeats. That would be a different story. More than likely his EKG would look similar, but his treatment might differ because the PACs would have been caused by something different. If the PACs occurred in clusters or with great frequency (10 per minute), and if the patient were taking digitalis, you might suspect the digitalis caused the PACs. Or, the patient could be having atrial bigeminy (a normal sinus beat that alternates with a PAC). Bigeminy is usually found in digitalized patients with a low serum potassium.

But the patient most likely to develop PACs is one with a history of heart disease, especially rheumatic carditis. This is because the rheumatic disease process irritates the atrial myocardium.

Whatever the cause of the PACs, the patient should be monitored for signs of other arrhythmias such as atrial tachycardias, which often follow PACs. Unless they produce other arrhythmias, PACs themselves are usually benign. Often they disappear without any treatment.

It should be obvious from this example that the treatment of PACs differs markedly, according to the clinical circumstances. The same is true of many other arrhythmias. As you read the following discussion of atrial arrhythmias, remember that the availability of a cardiac monitor by no means relieves you of the responsibility of making careful nursing observations. The EKG tracing only provides additional data to be interpreted in light of your patient's history and clinical appearance.

Three atrial tachycardias
Three arrhythmias are classified as atrial tachycardias. Each has a different mechanism, but all originate from atrial ectopic foci and have rates over 160 per minute.

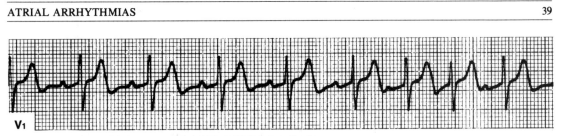

V₁

Figure 2 — PREMATURE ATRIAL CONTRACTION (PAC)

EKG Criteria:

1. Premature P wave may be lost in T wave or QRS complex.
2. P wave may have abnormal configuration (flat, slurred, notched, inverted, diphasic, or wide).
3. R-R interval of premature beat is shorter than normal.
4. P-R interval may be longer or (occasionally) shorter than normal, depending on location of P wave.
5. Pause following PAC is not usually compensatory (i.e., the beat following premature beat doesn't occur at normal time because SA node timing was disturbed).
6. QRS is normal, unless ventricular conduction is delayed or aberrant (follows a different pathway to ventricles).

Treatment

- Often no treatment is needed.
- If serum potassium is low, give I.V. potassium.
- Withhold digitalis if digitalis toxicity is the suspected cause of PACs.
- Give quinidine 200 mg, usually q.i.d., by mouth for patients with organic heart disease.
- Give propranolol if PACs occur in short runs of atrial tachycardia.

Pathway for atrial arrhythmias

Impulses for atrial arrhythmias originate outside the SA node, in either single or multiple ectopic foci.

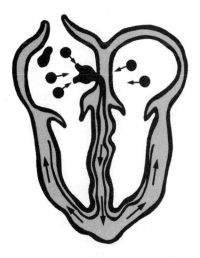

Paroxysmal atrial tachycardia (PAT) frequently occurs in normal, healthy persons. In such cases it is benign. But when it occurs in a cardiac patient or one who is critically ill, it can be a forerunner of a more serious ventricular arrhythmia.

PAT is a very rapid, regular heartbeat that begins suddenly and usually has been preceded by frequent PACs, one of which precipitates the tachycardia (see Figure 3). In some cases, the tachycardia is brief; in others it lasts for hours. Often PAT begins while the patient is asleep, and the rapid beating awakens him.

A physician may try one of two procedures to slow the rate. Either he'll ask the patient to take a deep breath and bear down (Valsalva's maneuver) or, he'll use carotid sinus pressure. Either method stimulates the vagus nerve and slows impulse production at the SA and AV nodes, causing atrial standstill and giving the SA node a chance to reestablish itself as the main pacemaker. Then normal sinus rhythm is restored.

When the atrial rate is exactly twice the ventricular rate, the patient is said to have PAT with 2:1 block. This is a common sign of toxicity in digitalized patients, who would require dosage adjustment to correct the arrhythmia.

Rapid rates can exhaust the patient, even those without organic disease. Therefore, you should watch the patient for signs of congestive heart failure. Be prepared to give an antiarrhythmic drug and diuretics as ordered, and to observe how they affect the patient and the arrhythmia.

Atrial flutter is an interesting arrhythmia, often misdiagnosed as PAT. As in PACs and PATs, the impulse comes from an atrial ectopic focus. Some cardiologists believe that the impulse derives from multiple ectopic foci ("circus movement"); others believe it derives from a single ectopic focus.

Atrial flutter rarely occurs in the absence of organic heart disease. Unless strictly controlled by the SA node, the atria love to go fast and are happy at 300. Actual atrial rates range from 220 to 350 beats per minute in patients with atrial flutter.

Because in this arrhythmia atrial activity is so chaotic, many of these impulses fail to pass through the AV node to the ventricles. Therefore, the atrial and ventricular rates differ greatly (e.g., 300 atrial, 75 ventricular for a ratio of 4:1). The failure of ventricles to keep pace is fortunate, since rapid ventricular rates pose a threat to the patient. A lower ratio between atrial and ventricular rates (e.g., 2:1 instead of 4:1) would more seriously threaten the patient because the ventricular rate would then be dangerously rapid.

In most cases of atrial flutter, the ventricular rhythm is very regular, but occasionally it is so irregular that you cannot establish a ratio between the atrial and ventricular rates (see Figure 4). An irregular ventricular rhythm often means the patient is getting ready to convert to atrial fibrillation, a favorable sign since atrial fibrillation responds more readily to drug treatment.

Most patients with atrial flutter respond to increased dosages of digitalis supplemented by propranolol (Inderal). This combination slows the impulses at the AV node, with the propranolol acting on the upper and lower nodal regions and digitalis affecting the midnodal region. As the ventricular rate slows, the atrial flutter converts to atrial fibrillation, which can be treated in turn with quinidine and maintenance dosages of digitalis. In some cases, the flutter reverts directly to normal sinus rhythm. Atrial flutter can also be treated by cardioversion or atrial pacing with a temporary pacemaker.

At times, you may not be able to distinguish on the rhythm strip between atrial flutter and the arrhythmia to be discussed next, atrial fib-

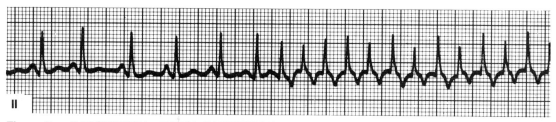

II

Figure 3 — PAROXYSMAL ATRIAL TACHYCARDIA (PAT)

EKG Criteria:

1. Ventricular rhythm is perfectly regular with atrial rate of 160 to 250.
2. QRS complex is usually narrow.
3. P waves may have an abnormal contour or be difficult to see in any of the 12 leads.
4. Onset is sudden, often initiated by PAC.

Treatment

- Apply Valsalva's maneuver.
- Apply carotid sinus pressure (only physicians do this).
- Give digitalis and diuretic to prevent congestive heart failure in prolonged tachycardia.

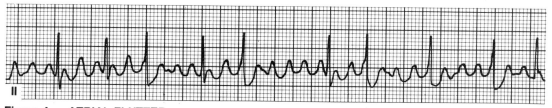

II

Figure 4 — ATRIAL FLUTTER

EKG Criteria:

I. P waves and T waves have merged to form sawtooth flutter waves (F waves).
2. QRS complex is usually narrow.
3. Atrial rate is between 250 and 350 beats per minute (usually 300/min.; determine rate by counting number of small squares between points of one sawtooth wave, then dividing into 1500).
4. Varying degrees of AV block (conduction) produce ventricular rates that are ½ to ¼ atrial rate, giving ratios of 2:1, 3:1, etc.
5. Ventricular rhythm, although usually regular, can be irregular because conduction ratio varies with each cycle.
6. All flutter waves are uniform in width and proceed through QRS complex without interfering with either rhythm.

Treatment

Administer or apply the following, either alone or in combination:

- Digitalis (unless flutter is due to digitalis toxicity)
- Propranolol
- Quinidine
- Diuretics, such as Lasix
- Elective cardioversion
- Temporary pacemaker

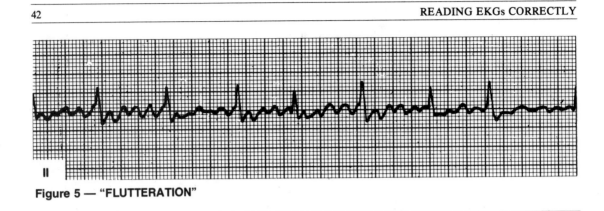

Figure 5 — "FLUTTERATION"

rillation (see Figure 5). These cases, representing either an impure flutter or a coarse fibrillation, are often referred to as "flutter-fib," "fibro-flutter," or, in our hospital, "flutteration." None of these words are standard medical terminology, but they do adequately describe the condition.

Atrial fibrillation is easily recognized because of its grossly irregular ventricular rhythm. As with the other atrial arrhythmias, the impulse originates in one or more irritable atrial ectopic areas. These ectopic foci discharge the impulses at atrial rates as high as 500 or more beats per minute. Such a rapid rate creates a chaotic baseline, of varying shapes and sizes (Figure 6). Unlike atrial flutter, in which the flutter waves are uniform, the fibrillatory (or f) waves cause the atrial rate to constantly change throughout the tracing.

With such excitable, irregular atrial activity, the ventricles respond only to those impulses that pass through the AV node. This is a sporadic occurrence, so in contrast to atrial flutter, the R-R interval of atrial fibrillation is very irregular, with no pattern to the irregularity. In those cases when the ventricular rate is too rapid, propranolol (Inderal) is added to the digitalis regimen to slow conduction through the AV node, thus slowing the ventricular response.

Some patients are admitted with the diagnosis of atrial fibrillation of unknown etiology. In many instances, despite the usual cardiac workup — 12-lead EKG, chest X-ray, cardiac enzyme and electrolyte studies, and continuous cardiac monitoring for several days — the etiology remains unknown. Such patients are usually discharged having had no dramatic treatment.

In fact, a large CCU will commonly have several patients in atrial fibrillation, each being treated differently. A striking example of this occurred in our hospital a while ago.

Same arrhythmia, different treatments

One afternoon, George R. and Helen E., both in their early 40s, were admitted to our CCU. Both had a preliminary diagnosis of atrial fibrillation with *uncontrolled* ventricular rates — his was about 150 (see Figure 7) and hers about 140 (see Figure 8). (Atrial fibrillation is considered *controlled* when the ventricular rate is below 100.) The admitting nurse noted moist rales in both patients' chests, but George was dyspneic; his breath sounds were coarse.

About an hour after admission, George was prepared for elective cardioversion. His atrial rate was 500 beats per minute, his ventricular rate, 150. He was given a Stat. I.V. push of digoxin, 0.25 mg, with little effect on his heart rate. He was also given nasal oxygen at 5 L/min for the dyspnea and Lasix, 20 mg I.V., for the

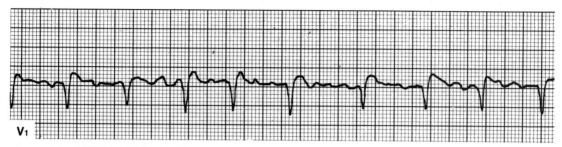

V₁

Figure 6 — ATRIAL FIBRILLATION

EKG Criteria:
1. Ventricular rhythm is completely irregular, with no pattern to irregularity.
2. Atrial fibrillatory (f) waves may be superimposed on T waves.
3. Atrial rate (determined as in atrial flutter) is between 350 and 500 beats per minute (could go as high as 700 beats per minute).
4. No P-R interval is visible.
5. QRS is usually narrow unless conduction is delayed in ventricles.

Treatment
Administer or apply any of the following, alone or in combination:
• Digitalis, quinidine, or propranolol to slow ventricular rate and to convert to normal sinus rhythm.
• Diuretics for congestive heart failure.
• Elective cardioversion.
• Temporary pacemaker for low ventricular rates due to block.

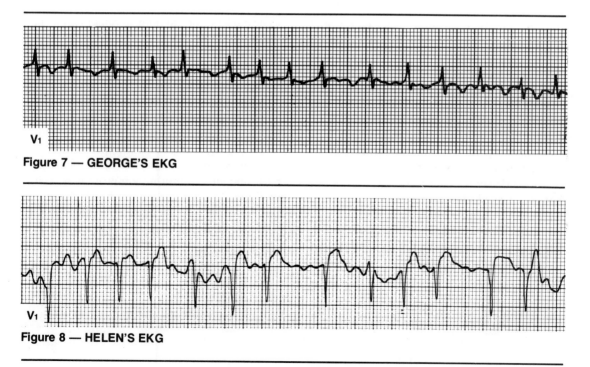

V₁

Figure 7 — GEORGE'S EKG

V₁

Figure 8 — HELEN'S EKG

rales, which were becoming more pronounced. His response to the diuretic was fair.

Meanwhile, Helen was also given digoxin, 0.25 mg Stat. I.V., and Lasix 10 mg I.M., to slow her heart rate and prevent congestive heart failure. An additional 0.25 mg dose of digoxin was given I.M. 2 hours later because her ventricular rate remained above 100 beats per minute. Quinidine, 200 mg by mouth q.i.d., and oxygen p.r.n. for dyspnea were also ordered.

Helen's urine output increased in response to the diuretic. After the first dose of digoxin, her ventricular rate slowed to 110; after the second dose, to 90. Her atrial fibrillation was thus considered controlled.

Why were these two patients, with the same arrhythmia, treated so differently? Primarily, because their medical histories were vastly different.

George had a history of two previous myocardial infarctions, the last one complicated by severe congestive heart failure and episodes of PVCs. Because his myocardium was severely damaged, his increasingly irregular heart rate threatened to bring on congestive heart failure and a more lethal arrhythmia.

After two shocks of 50 w/sec each, the cardioversion restored his heart to a normal sinus rhythm of 86 beats per minute. He was then given digoxin, 0.25 mg by mouth b.i.d., and his daily Lasix dose was increased to 20 mg by mouth b.i.d. He was observed for a week and then discharged, doing well.

Helen had been hospitalized several times for evaluation and treatment of mitral stenosis. Her ventricular myocardium was undamaged,

so we knew we had time to observe her and could treat her more conservatively. Besides, in patients with mitral stenosis and atrial fibrillation, cardioversion increases the risk of an embolus from left atrial clots (commonly found in patients with mitral stenosis).

She was hospitalized for 3 weeks. She underwent successful open-heart surgery for her mitral stenosis. When discharged she still had atrial fibrillation with a ventricular rate of 76 — not a serious problem for her. Cardioversion was not attempted postoperatively because a patient with long-standing fibrillation with mitral stenosis isn't likely to return to sinus rhythm.

Upon discharge, Helen was doing well on medication — digoxin, 0.25 mg, and hydrochlorothiazide, 50 mg daily. She was also taking quinidine, 200 mg q.i.d., to minimize irritability of the myocardium and prevent any further tachycardia.

The most important thing to remember is that even a confirmed diagnosis of an arrhythmia means nothing by itself. The seriousness of an arrhythmia can be judged only in the context of its meaning to the patient.

This is where you, the nurse, come in. Who can better judge the patient's changes in condition? You know how the patient looks, and if there were any changes in his appearance. You have access to his history, his care plans, his chart, and all the information pertaining to his condition. You must consider all of this information before you can determine what action, if any, is required when changes occur in the patient's rhythm strip or in his condition.

SKILLCHECK 4

The two hallmarks of atrial arrhythmias are that their P waves *usually* are absent (as with atrial fibrillation) or abnormal (ectopic, as with PAT or atrial flutter), and that they *usually,* though not always, are rapid. As you identify the following EKGs, check to see whether they meet these standards. (Remember that, even though they may not, they still may be atrial arrhythmias.)

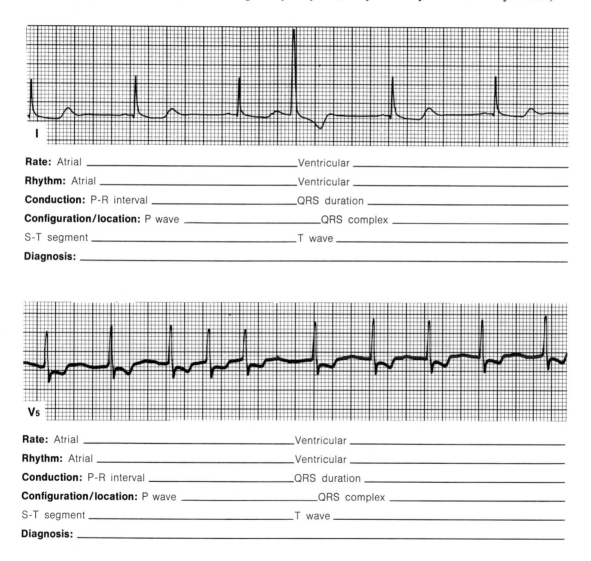

Rate: Atrial _____Ventricular _____

Rhythm: Atrial _____Ventricular _____

Conduction: P-R interval _____QRS duration _____

Configuration/location: P wave _____QRS complex _____

S-T segment _____T wave _____

Diagnosis: _____

Rate: Atrial _____Ventricular _____

Rhythm: Atrial _____Ventricular _____

Conduction: P-R interval _____QRS duration _____

Configuration/location: P wave _____QRS complex _____

S-T segment _____T wave _____

Diagnosis: _____

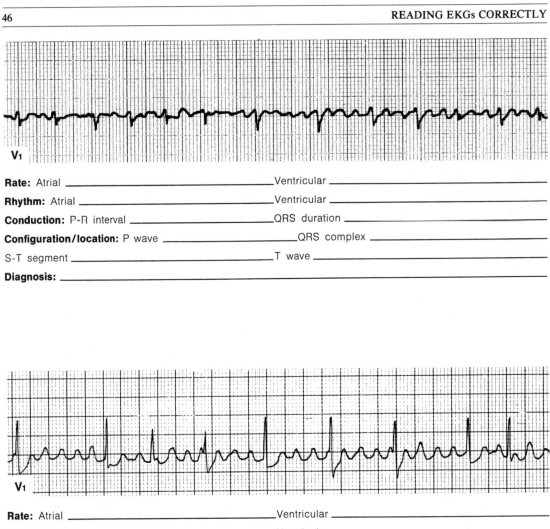

V₁

Rate: Atrial _____ Ventricular _____

Rhythm: Atrial _____ Ventricular _____

Conduction: P-R interval _____ QRS duration _____

Configuration/location: P wave _____ QRS complex _____

S-T segment _____ T wave _____

Diagnosis: _____

V₁

Rate: Atrial _____ Ventricular _____

Rhythm: Atrial _____ Ventricular _____

Conduction: P-R interval _____ QRS duration _____

Configuration/location: P wave _____ QRS complex _____

S-T segment _____ T wave _____

Diagnosis: _____

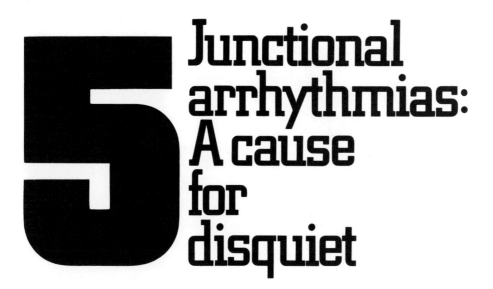

5 Junctional arrhythmias: A cause for disquiet

Watching an EKG tracing emerge from the machine, you sometimes feel your anxiety rising. Being a professional, you don't let it show. But you're also human; you cannot avoid reacting emotionally to evidence on that rhythm strip suggesting that your patient is a lot sicker than anybody had imagined.

In the next three chapters, we'll be discussing arrhythmias capable of raising a nurse's anxiety level: junctional arrhythmias, AV blocks, and ventricular arrhythmias and bundle branch blocks. All contrast with sinus and atrial arrhythmias, which, except for atrial flutter, can and often do appear in healthy people. Junctional arrhythmias, AV blocks, ventricular arrhythmias, and bundle branch blocks hardly ever occur in healthy people and almost always are serious.

Even though junctional arrhythmias are generally regarded as the least dangerous of this group, they are serious and call for prompt treatment.

What causes junctional arrhythmias?
The SA node is the heart's normal pacemaker. However, the AV node takes over this role in certain cases of organic heart disease, atrial ischemia, a myocardial infarction, or overdigitalization.

When the AV node assumes the pacemaker role, *junctional arrhythmias* result. The impulse originating in the AV node travels first to the ventricles, then rebounds to stimulate the atria. Called *retrograde conduction,* this abnormal mechanism in which the impulse reaches the ventricles before reaching the atria may diminish cardiac output, especially when the ventricular rate is very slow or very rapid.

Consequently, junctional arrhythmias are serious. They usually occur in patients who have organic heart disease and may lead to congestive heart failure.

Premature beats. If the AV node takes over as the dominant pacemaker for only one beat, it is called a *junctional premature beat* or a

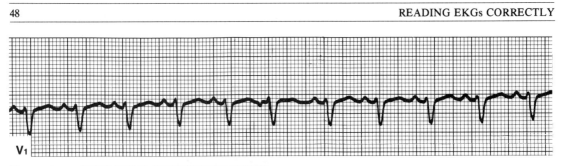

Figure 1 — JUNCTIONAL PREMATURE BEATS

EKG Criteria:

1. R-R interval of premature beat is shorter than patient's normal interval.
2. P-R interval is short (less than 0.12 seconds).
3. P wave inverts in II, III, and aVF and is upright in aVR and aVL.
4. P wave may be lost in QRS or follow QRS and be inverted.

Treatment

● Give K+ supplement if indicated.
● Give quinidine or Pronestyl.

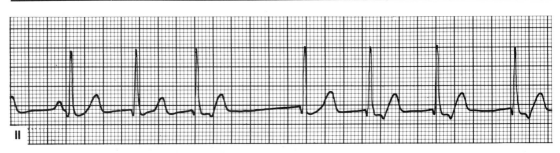
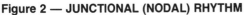

Figure 2 — JUNCTIONAL (NODAL) RHYTHM

EKG Criteria:

1. P wave precedes QRS complex but P-R interval is shorter than 0.11 seconds. (P wave could be inverted in leads II and III.)
2. Or P wave, lost in QRS complex, is not visible.
3. Or P wave follows QRS complex and is inverted (retrograde conduction).
4. QRS duration is normal unless conduction is aberrant.
5. Ventricular rate is between 40 and 60 beats per minute.

Treatment

● Give diuretic to prevent or control congestive heart failure.
● Give diphenylhydantoin (Dilantin) I.V. or I.M.
● Insert temporary pacemaker if cardiac output is poor.

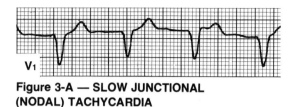

Figure 3-A — SLOW JUNCTIONAL (NODAL) TACHYCARDIA

EKG Criteria:
1. Same P wave location and QRS complex as in junctional rhythm.
2. Ventricular rate is 60-100 (slow) or 100-220 (rapid). (Rapid junctional tachycardia of sudden onset is paroxysmal junctional tachycardia.)

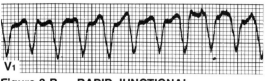

Figure 3-B — RAPID JUNCTIONAL (NODAL) TACHYCARDIA

Treatment
- If digitalis toxicity is the cause (likely in paroxysmal junctional tachycardia), withhold dosage and give diuretic to prevent congestive heart failure.
- Give propranolol.
- Give diphenylhydantoin (Dilantin).
- Give potassium chloride I.V. with I.V. fluids ordered.
- Initiate cardioversion.

premature nodal contraction (PNC). It can be caused by an excess of digitalis or an excess of quinidine.

You can differentiate between an atrial premature beat and a junctional premature beat by the location of the P wave. In a PAC, the R-R interval is shorter than normal and the P wave may appear closer to or as part of the T wave, making the P-R interval longer. In a PNC (Figure 1), the R-R interval also is shorter than normal. But the P wave may be closer to, be lost in, or follow the QRS complex, making the P-R interval short (less than 0.12 seconds).

Sometimes, though, the P wave may be so indistinct that you can't tell whether it's a PAC or a PNC. What then? That's when you have to make a judgment based on the patient's history and diagnosis. Does he have rheumatic carditis, for example — a common cause of PACs? Or does he have organic heart disease — common in patients with PNCs? Is his serum potassium level low, as it often is with PACs? Answers to these questions should give you a clue to the problem.

Still, there are times when the answers don't help — no one can determine whether a patient

has PACs or PNCs. All that can be said for certain is that the impulse originates above the bifurcation of the bundle of His. Since the exact origin of these beats is unknown, they are called *supraventricular premature beats.*

Whatever the origin of the premature beat, you must stay alert for other developing arrhythmias. If any arise, immediately report them to the doctor. If the patient's serum potassium is low, the doctor may order an I.V. potassium supplement; often, that's enough to eliminate the premature beats. If the patient has ventricular damage (e.g., myocardial infarction), the doctor may order quinidine or Pronestyl by mouth to quell or prevent ventricular irritability.

Nodal rhythms. If the AV node takes over as the dominant pacemaker for a succession of beats, the patient is in *nodal rhythm* or *nodal tachycardia.* Usually, the AV node can initiate impulses of from 40 to 60 beats per minute, the so-called *junctional* (or *nodal*) *rhythm* (Figure 2). A junctional rhythm of more than 60 beats per minute is called *junctional tachycardia* (see Figures 3-A and 3-B). Junctional tachycardia may be either slow (under 100 beats per minute) or rapid (over 100 beats per minute). A junc-

The terms "nodal," "junctional," and "AV junctional" arrhythmias all refer to arrhythmias originating in the AV node.

tional tachycardia of sudden onset, called *paroxysmal junctional tachycardia,* usually indicates digitalis toxicity (150 to 220 beats per minute).

The terms "nodal," "junctional," and "AV junctional" arrhythmia are used interchangeably; all refer to an arrhythmia originating in the AV node. To further complicate terminology, many electrocardiographers and textbooks refer to a specific section of the AV node in diagnosing an arrhythmia. Anatomically, the AV node is divided into upper, middle, and lower nodal regions. The upper nodal region borders on the atria; the lower, on the bundle of His. (This entire region is also referred to as the junctional region.)

An upper nodal arrhythmia can be identified by a short P-R interval, with an inverted P wave preceding the QRS complex. In a midnodal arrhythmia, the P wave may be "riding" or entirely lost in the QRS complex. A low nodal arrhythmia is identified by an inverted P wave following the QRS complex. At times, it's extremely difficult to determine whether the arrhythmia, like a single premature junctional contraction, is derived from an impulse originating in the low atrial region or the upper nodal region. Although in such cases the point of origin is not precisely known, it is known to be located above the ventricles; hence the resulting disturbance or arrhythmia is classified simply as a *supraventricular arrhythmia.*

A case in point
Whatever the specific origin of impulse, a junctional arrhythmia poses real danger to the patient, as this example shows.

Rosemary P., a 35-year-old mother of three, came to our ICU immediately after her third operation for mitral valve disease. This time the surgeon implanted a Starr-Edwards mitral valve prosthesis, and we hoped it would see her through many good years. Since most of us had

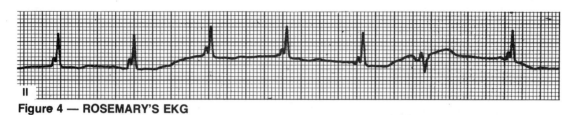

II

Figure 4 — ROSEMARY'S EKG

been on the unit when Rosemary had had her previous operations, we considered her almost part of the family. We wanted to make this postop period as easy as possible for her.

Although concerned about the usual postop heart surgery complications (e.g., shock, hemorrhage, stroke from emboli), we were even more concerned about the possibility of a serious arrhythmia. We'd have been surprised if Rosemary had maintained the normal sinus rhythm she had upon return from the O.R. Like most mitral patients, she'd had atrial fibrillation for years, so we expected her to revert to it soon.

Midmorning of Rosemary's first postop day, her rhythm on the monitor changed abruptly to a slow junctional tachycardia, with premature ventricular contractions (PVCs) close to the T wave. We did a Stat. EKG to confirm the junctional pacing, then looked for better P waves, especially in leads II and V₁.

A portion of Rosemary's rhythm strip is shown in Figure 4. Can you analyze it? Compare your analysis with the criteria for junctional rhythm and junctional tachycardia (Figures 2, 3-A, and 3-B).

Notice how close the P waves are to the QRS complex and how short the P-R interval is. Clearly, the impulse could not be coming from the SA node. The PVC's proximity to the T wave of the preceding beat is another danger sign, which we'll discuss in Chapter 7.

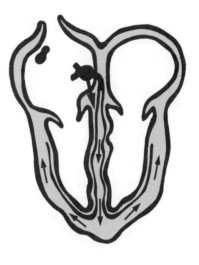

Pathway for junctional arrhythmias

When the AV node assumes the pacemaker role, junctional arrhythmias result.

What caused Rosemary's arrhythmia? We suspected digitalis might have caused it. Since surgery she had been given a total of only 1.0 mg of digoxin — not an excessive dosage for a postop patient with mitral valve disease. However, if hypokalemia were present, digitalis toxicity could still have been responsible. Another likely cause was the heart's inflammation and edema resulting from the recent surgery.

Besides keeping a close watch on her EKG, we watched Rosemary for signs of congestive heart failure, listening to her chest for moist rales and carefully checking her fluid intake and output as well as vital signs.

As a precaution we withheld further digitalis. We added 40 mEq of potassium chloride to the day's I.V. fluids (a total of 1,000 cc) because her serum potassium was 3.9. Although this is not dangerously low, hypokalemia could have contributed to the arrhythmia.

Because of Rosemary's cardiac history and the PVCs, we started Pronestyl (procainamide), 1 Gm in 500 cc of 5% dextrose in water, by piggyback I.V., slowly, and gave quinidine, 200 mg q6h, by mouth. The Pronestyl and quinidine combination quieted both the atrial and ventricular myocardial irritability, and the PVCs soon disappeared. The junctional rate held steady at 72 — a slow junctional tachycardia.

Midafternoon of the second postop day, Rosemary converted to atrial fibrillation with a ventricular rate of 84. The PVCs had not recurred, so we discontinued the Pronestyl early that evening but continued the quinidine until after discharge. (Quinidine is commonly used prophylactically on patients like Rosemary.) We restarted digoxin, 0.25 mg, on the third postop day, and Rosemary had no further arrhythmias during the remainder of her hospitalization.

In one respect, Rosemary was fortunate. Her ventricular rate with the junctional arrhythmia never exceeded 72. In an arrhythmia caused by digitalis toxicity, the ventricular rate could have increased to as high as 220 beats per minute. Such rapid rates greatly decrease cardiac output, which could be fatal to a patient in Rosemary's condition.

Although not needed in Rosemary's case, in many cases propranolol is used to reverse paroxysmal junctional tachycardia. If this fails, cardioversion may be tried.

SKILLCHECK 5

As we've said, sometimes it is impossible to distinguish a PNC from a PAC or to determine whether a nodal arrhythmia originates in the upper nodal region or the low atrial region. In those cases, you'll have to rely on other information to assess the EKG tracing, or simply describe it as a supraventricular arrhythmia. In other cases, though, the P-R interval will give you the clue you need to make an assessment. Pay particular attention to the P-R interval in the following tracings to help you identify them.

Rate: Atrial _____ Ventricular _____

Rhythm: Atrial _____ Ventricular _____

Conduction: P-R interval _____ QRS duration _____

Configuration/location: P wave _____ QRS complex _____

S-T segment _____ T wave _____

Diagnosis: _____

Rate: Atrial _____ Ventricular _____

Rhythm: Atrial _____ Ventricular _____

Conduction: P-R interval _____ QRS duration _____

Configuration/location: P wave _____ QRS complex _____

S-T segment _____ T wave _____

Diagnosis: _____

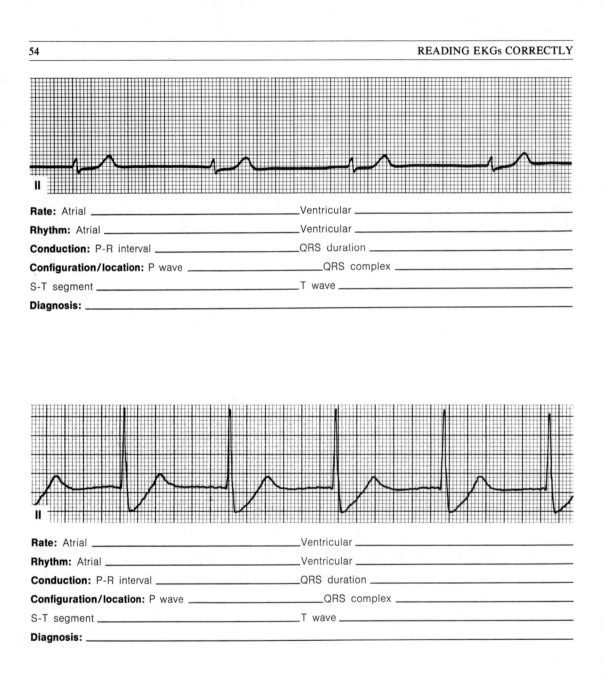

Rate: Atrial _____ Ventricular _____

Rhythm: Atrial _____ Ventricular _____

Conduction: P-R interval _____ QRS duration _____

Configuration/location: P wave _____ QRS complex _____

S-T segment _____ T wave _____

Diagnosis: _____

Rate: Atrial _____ Ventricular _____

Rhythm: Atrial _____ Ventricular _____

Conduction: P-R interval _____ QRS duration _____

Configuration/location: P wave _____ QRS complex _____

S-T segment _____ T wave _____

Diagnosis: _____

6 AV blocks: The value of a suspicious mind

By now you should realize that EKG interpretation takes a lot more than a few technical skills. No doubt you've found it takes something closer to the artistry of a practiced sleuth: a sharp eye for detail and the persistence to explore all possible interpretations. But more than that, it takes a suspicious mind — a developed instinct to suspect the worst possible explanation first and then to try to disprove it. If your worst suspicion proves incorrect, you can still go on to test for less serious conditions. But if your worst suspicion proves correct, you'll be on top of the situation and have plenty of time to correct it.

The value of a suspicious mind underlies all EKG interpretation, but it is especially important with AV blocks. As many tragic stories attest, too often nurses glance only at the monitor and so mistake these dangerous arrhythmias for a sinus bradycardia or a sinus arrhythmia. They fail to check the rhythm strip. So, while they go on to examine the rhythm strip of another patient with "a serious problem," the

patient with the dangerous AV block slips into congestive heart failure. Efforts to resuscitate fail. Such tragedies could easily be avoided if only nurses would remember to suspect the worst first and to thoroughly check their suspicions.

AV block

Any conduction disturbance in the heart is referred to as a block. The most common are AV blocks, a conduction delay in the AV node, which are classified as: first-degree AV block, second-degree AV block — Mobitz Type I (or Wenckebach) and Mobitz Type II — and third-degree AV block (complete heart block).

We can also classify blocks according to cause. Chemical blocks are caused by excessive doses of such drugs as digitalis or quinidine. Pathologic blocks are caused by myocardial infarction or degeneration of conduction tissue due to age. Mechanical blocks are most apt to be caused by inadvertently placing a suture through the AV node during open heart surgery,

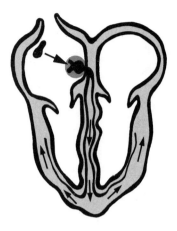

Pathway of AV blocks

Although the impulse originates in the SA node, an abnormality in the AV node blocks it.

resulting in impaired atrioventricular conduction. Physiologic blocks following open heart surgery are caused by manipulation or by edema in the nodal region resulting in damage (usually temporary) to nodal tissue.

Sometimes the AV node itself is refractory to an impulse — it doesn't or can't permit the impulse to pass directly through it. Instead the impulse must reach the ventricles by traveling around the AV node instead of through it (aberrant conduction).

As with arrhythmias discussed earlier, you can gain insight into the location and type of block from the EKG, but to decide on appropriate treatment, you must know the cause of the block, and the patient's response to it. You might have two patients on your unit with second-degree AV block. One might require immediate treatment, the other only close observation. What treatment, if any, is required would depend primarily on the deterioration in cardiac output resulting from the arrhythmia.

An asymptomatic patient is apt to require only observation; very likely no symptoms will develop and no treatment may be needed. On the other hand, the onset of syncope or convulsions would point to severe block with a very slow ventricular rate, requiring immediate treatment. The treatment might consist of temporary pacing with a demand pacemaker to improve cardiac function. The temporary pacing will give you time to observe how much pacing your patient requires, to decide when and if he will require permanent pacing, and to teach him how to live with a permanent pacemaker if it's needed.

A less aggressive treatment for patients with low output blocks is atropine, which increases atrial contractility by speeding the rate of the sinus node. If the AV node is not too badly damaged, the atropine improves conduction of impulses to the ventricles, thereby improving cardiac output.

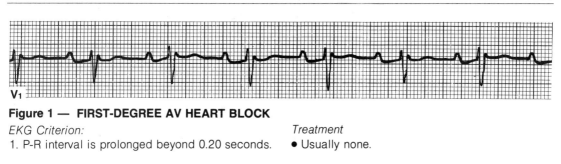

Figure 1 — FIRST-DEGREE AV HEART BLOCK

EKG Criterion:
1. P-R interval is prolonged beyond 0.20 seconds.

Treatment
• Usually none.

For some patients isoproterenol (Isuprel) may be used to improve cardiac output. However, using isoproterenol is riskier than atropine because in many cases it increases myocardial irritability, predisposing to PVCs, or perhaps ventricular tachycardia.

First-degree AV block
The most common conduction disturbance, first-degree AV block, can occur in apparently healthy persons as well as in those with diseased hearts. First-degree block is usually clinically insignificant; certainly it is considered less dangerous than the other types of blocks.

Chronic degeneration of the conduction system causes first-degree block in many elderly patients without evidence of heart disease. Antiarrhythmic drugs such as quinidine and procainamide are another cause of first-degree block. In children, acute rheumatic fever may be the cause; indeed, first-degree block may be the earliest sign of the disease.

In first-degree AV block, impulses are conducted normally from the SA node through the atria but are delayed when they reach the AV node. The block can be recognized on the EKG: each P wave is followed by a QRS complex, but the P-R interval is prolonged — 0.20 seconds or

longer (see Figure 1). Although generally constant, the P-R intervals may vary slightly if the heart rate changes significantly. In some instances, the P-R interval may be as long as 0.70 to 0.80 seconds. Then the P wave may be fused with the preceding T wave, resembling an AV nodal rhythm. When the P-R interval is exceptionally long, you should also suspect hidden P waves, which may signify second-degree AV block. You'll need to carefully inspect the full 12-lead EKG to detect the P wave before you can make a diagnosis.

By itself, first-degree AV block does not significantly affect cardiac output. But if a patient's myocardium is already severely damaged, the block may advance to a more serious state because of the damage to or near the conduction system.

Second-degree AV block
There are two types of second-degree AV block: Mobitz Type I (or Wenckebach) and Mobitz Type II. Both types are characterized by occasional dropped ventricular beats. On the EKG this will show up as a series of normal cycles, then a P wave appears without a QRS complex. Dropped beats mean that the impulse was conducted through the atria, but its passage

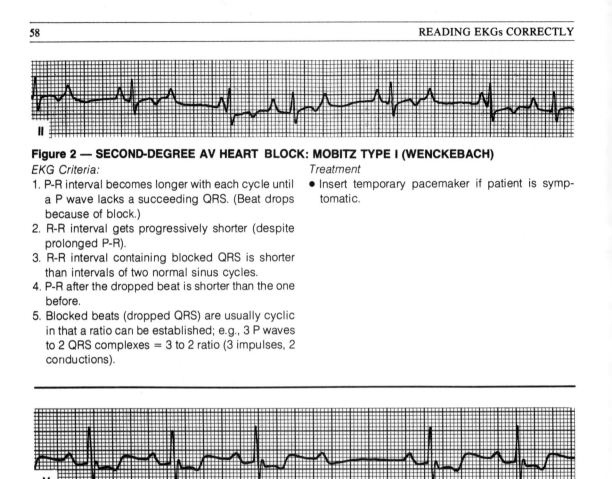

Figure 2 — SECOND-DEGREE AV HEART BLOCK: MOBITZ TYPE I (WENCKEBACH)

EKG Criteria:

1. P-R interval becomes longer with each cycle until a P wave lacks a succeeding QRS. (Beat drops because of block.)
2. R-R interval gets progressively shorter (despite prolonged P-R).
3. R-R interval containing blocked QRS is shorter than intervals of two normal sinus cycles.
4. P-R after the dropped beat is shorter than the one before.
5. Blocked beats (dropped QRS) are usually cyclic in that a ratio can be established; e.g., 3 P waves to 2 QRS complexes = 3 to 2 ratio (3 impulses, 2 conductions).

Treatment

- Insert temporary pacemaker if patient is symptomatic.

Figure 3 — SECOND-DEGREE AV HEART BLOCK: MOBITZ TYPE II

EKG Criteria:

1. P-R interval is constant.
2. QRS complex is periodically dropped after a P wave. (Beat is dropped because of block.)

Treatment

- Insert temporary pacemaker and, eventually, permanent pacemaker.

through the AV node was blocked. Generally, in second-degree AV block the AV conduction ratio is 3:2 or 4:3, indicating that two out of three or three out of four impulses are conducted to the ventricles.

The Mobitz Type I (Wenckebach) AV block occurs most frequently in patients who have an inferior wall myocardial infarction or digitalis toxicity. Often a transient arrhythmia, it may also be caused by acute rheumatic fever, electrolyte imbalance, vagal stimulation, and occasionally by quinidine or procainamide therapy.

In the Mobitz Type I block, the P-R interval is normal or even short to begin with, but with each cycle it gets longer and longer until finally a QRS complex is dropped. Then the cycle begins again with a normal or slightly short P-R interval (see Figure 2).

Here's what happens: Diseased conducting tissues of the AV node become fatigued more easily than normal tissues. Conduction of each impulse causes greater fatigue, so each sinus impulse is conducted more and more slowly (prolonging the P-R interval). Finally, the tissues become so fatigued that they are not able to conduct the sinus impulse at all; passage through the AV node is thus blocked. But this also gives the AV node a chance to rest, so it can conduct the next impulse in the normal time.

Less frequently, a Mobitz Type I block may have only one nonconducted P wave between long periods of normally conducted P waves. Then the progression of the prolonged P-R interval may be so slight that it will be difficult to detect.

In Mobitz Type I block, the ventricular rhythm is slightly irregular because the R-R intervals become progressively shorter despite the prolonged P-R interval. The atrial rhythm, however, usually remains regular.

If the patient is asymptomatic, the prognosis usually is good for this Mobitz Type I second-degree block. Generally, it doesn't significantly affect cardiac output because the ventricular rate remains nearly normal.

Mobitz Type II AV block is less common than Mobitz Type I, but is also more serious, occurring mostly in patients with acute myocardial infarction or severe coronary artery disease. Often, it progresses to third-degree or complete block, requiring permanent pacing.

Type II resembles Type I in that both are characterized by dropped QRS complexes, but in Type II the P-R and P-P intervals do not vary. In other words, the dropped beat occurs completely without warning, in contrast to the prolonged P-R interval that signals an impending dropped beat in Mobitz Type I block. Figure 3 shows a Mobitz Type II 4:3 block.

In either type of second-degree block, the seriousness can be determined by the width of the QRS complex. If the QRS is narrow, the block is higher in the AV node and is less dangerous to the patient. If the QRS is wide, the block is farther down in the conduction system — usually below the bundle of His or near the bundle branches. This indicates seriously damaged cardiac tissue, often including the bundle branches; it is much more dangerous to the patient (e.g., it could produce Stokes-Adams syndrome). Hence, permanent pacing usually is required.

Another type of second-degree AV block that must be considered separately is 2:1 AV block. In 2:1 AV block, every second sinus or atrial impulse is blocked; i.e., every other QRS complex is dropped. Therefore, each QRS complex is associated with two P waves. If 2:1 block occurs by itself, it's usually impossible to determine whether it is Mobitz Type I or II because you cannot determine the P-R interval. Since you cannot determine if it is prolonged, you'll have to observe the rhythm and the patient for signs of improvement or deterioration. With that information you should be able to classify the block.

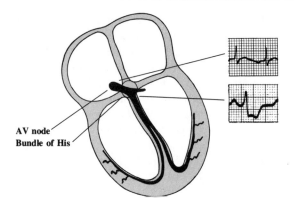

AV node
Bundle of His

Location of heart block as indicated by QRS

If the block occurs high in the junctional region (AV node), the QRS complex will usually be narrow. If the block occurs lower in the junctional region (bundle of His), the QRS will usually be wide. This conduction delay inhibits ventricular function and increases the likelihood of ventricular arrhythmias.

Third-degree AV block

In third-degree AV block (complete heart block), the atria and ventricles act independently of each other, each producing its own impulses. This occurs because a complete block at the AV junction prevents all the impulses produced in the SA node from passing through to the ventricles. So, the ventricles must initiate their own impulse; the ventricular rate is then determined by the block's location and the origin of the subsidiary impulse.

If the block occurs high in the AV node, the subsidiary pacemaker will be below the blocked area but still high in the AV node (above the bundle of His). The ventricular rate will be 45 to 60 beats per minute — slightly slower than normal sinus rhythm. In these instances the QRS will usually be narrow.

If the block occurs lower in the AV junction, the subsidiary pacemaker will be below the bundle of His, perhaps in the bundle branches, and the ventricular rate will be between 30 and 40 beats per minute. Here the QRS will usually be wide. These rates of less than 40 beats per minute are also called *idioventricular rhythms* since they arise in lower portions of the AV node or the ventricles. Rates this slow impair cardiac output and thus pose a danger to the patient.

In patients with third-degree block, the atrial rate is faster than the ventricular rate (see Figure 4). The atrial impulse may originate in the SA node, producing normal sinus rhythm, or it may originate in an atrial ectopic focus, producing atrial tachycardia, atrial flutter, or atrial fibrillation.

In some cases complete block is due to digitalis toxicity. Such arrhythmias are likely to be transient, and the ventricular rate is likely to be rapid enough to prevent syncope or congestive heart failure. Beyond discontinuing digitalis and observing for signs of impaired cardiac output, many patients require no treatment; others require a temporary pacemaker.

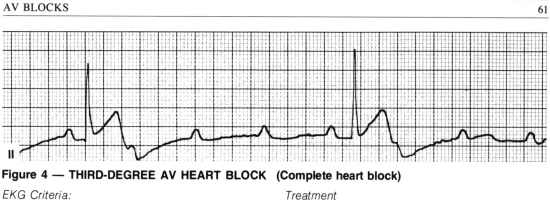

Figure 4 — THIRD-DEGREE AV HEART BLOCK **(Complete heart block)**

EKG Criteria:
1. Atrial and ventricular rates differ. Atrial rate is fast; ventricular rate is slow.
2. P waves are not related to QRS complexes; i.e., they do not indicate ventricular contraction from a sinus beat because impulse is not conducted to ventricles (AV dissociation).
3. P-R interval varies.

Treatment
- Insert permanent pacemaker if necessary.
- Stop digitalis if block is due to toxicity.

In other cases, third-degree AV block may be congenital — or it may be caused by acute rheumatic fever, acute myocardial infarction, or diffuse fibrosis throughout the conduction system. It may also occur after open-heart surgery, especially in patients with septal defects.

If the block is congenital, it usually does not cause symptoms and no pacing is required despite the slow ventricular rates. The reason for this is not well understood. In contrast, an acquired complete block almost always produces symptoms, such as Stokes-Adams syncope, severe congestive heart failure, and ventricular irritability (PVCs or runs of ventricular tachycardia).

Complete block in a patient with acute myocardial infarction may be either transient or permanent, depending on the amount of myocardial damage and the subsidiary pacemaker site. For example, if a patient with acute inferior myocardial infarction develops complete block with a ventricular rate exceeding 50 beats per minute and has no signs of congestive heart failure, he may only require monitoring and, possibly, small doses of atropine. If the patient develops a ventricular rate below 40 beats per minute, hypotension, or congestive heart failure, a temporary pacemaker may be inserted. Normal AV conduction usually returns within 5 to 7 days. But slow heart rates predispose to PVCs (rule of bigeminy) and runs of ventricular tachycardia.

In contrast, a patient with anterior wall myocardial infarction who develops complete block usually does develop symptoms: often either syncope or congestive heart failure. Because the myocardium is severely damaged, a permanent pacemaker usually must be inserted. Even so, damage to the anterior wall implies a poor prognosis, as illustrated by the following example.

AV block resulting from infarction
While at work Jim C., a 42-year-old advertising executive, had a sudden, sharp, stabbing pain in his chest that radiated down his left arm. He was

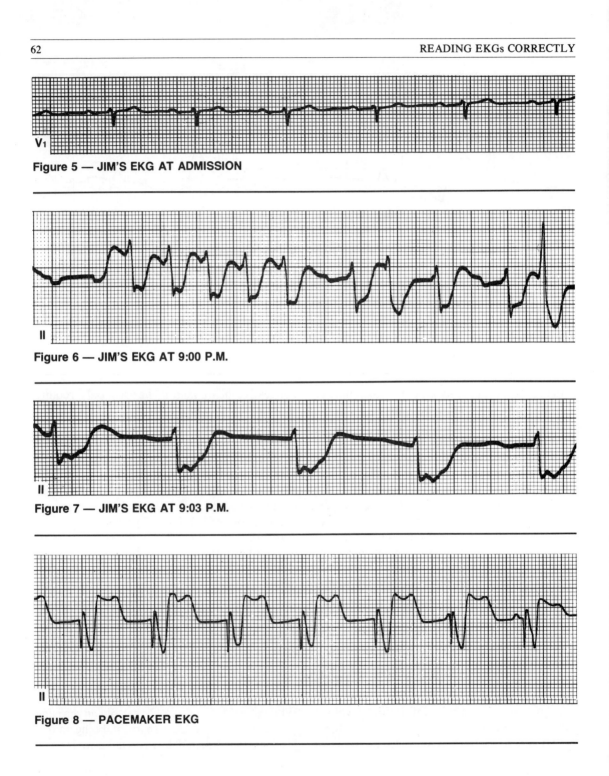

Figure 5 — JIM'S EKG AT ADMISSION

Figure 6 — JIM'S EKG AT 9:00 P.M.

Figure 7 — JIM'S EKG AT 9:03 P.M.

Figure 8 — PACEMAKER EKG

brought to our hospital by the police emergency rescue squad. Within minutes after his arrival, he was admitted to our coronary care unit.

Jim's history was typical. He had a high-pressure job and frequently suffered bouts of chest discomfort, fatigue, and indigestion. He carried a supply of Alka Seltzer and Tums with him at all times. His family had a history of coronary disease, hypertension, and diabetes, and Jim himself was a heavy smoker, overweight, and hypertensive.

Suspecting a myocardial infarction, we gave him a complete medical workup, including laboratory and X-ray studies. Meanwhile, we treated him as an MI patient according to our CCU routine.

We ran a Stat. 12-lead EKG and initiated cardiac monitoring. We also started an I.V., drew blood for measuring cardiac enzymes and arterial blood gases and for routine studies. We started nasal oxygen and gave him Demerol, 100 mg, for the recurring pain. Looking at Figure 5, can you analyze Jim's rhythm strip?

Jim had a slow sinus rhythm at a rate of 60 beats per minute and his P-R interval was slightly prolonged at 0.24 seconds, indicating first-degree AV block. The S-T segment is slightly elevated and the T wave is changing shape indicating anterior wall ischemia. These EKG changes plus his pain and history led us to suspect that Jim would soon progress to an anterior wall infarction. We watched closely for additional arrhythmias (e.g., PVCs or a higher degree of block). We knew that the slow rate could cause congestive heart failure, but it had not yet caused any apparent ill effects.

We monitored Jim's EKG, fluid balance, vital signs, breath sounds, and clinical picture. We looked for signs of congestive heart failure or deterioration in cardiac status.

That evening about 7:00, Jim's QRS complex widened to 0.16 seconds, but his heart rate was 60 beats per minute. The P-R interval increased to 0.32 seconds. Then everything seemed to happen at once. As Jim's nightmare began, so did ours.

At 9:00, Jim developed a short run of ventricular tachycardia (Figure 6) quickly followed by complete heart block with a ventricular rate of 44 (Figure 7). Conduction to the ventricles had deteriorated and his condition was critical. He became diaphoretic and restless. His blood pressure fell to 90/60. His urine output decreased. Then he began to have frequent PVCs. After a lidocaine bolus of 50 mg, we started a lidocaine drip. However, with AV block lidocaine must be administered cautiously because it may further increase the degree of block, even though it suppresses the PVCs.

Jim was in shock. A temporary demand pacemaker set for 75 beats per minute was inserted. The pacemaker fired continuously to maintain this rate. (Since pacemakers are common treatment for some arrhythmias, you should be able to recognize the distinctive EKG features they produce — a widened QRS and a pacemaker spike in or before the QRS complex. Figure 8 illustrates these.) Jim's PVCs disappeared, his blood pressure rose to 110/70, and his general condition improved. Although we could have given him Isuprel, Aramine, epinephrine, or Levophed to raise his blood pressure, the pacemaker seemed best at the time because of the severity of shock. For the next several hours, Jim's condition remained stable and he rested.

The next morning, shortly after the change of shift, Jim developed intense chest pain and, in quick succession PVCs, ventricular fibrillation, and cardiac arrest. Our efforts to resuscitate him failed.

We obtained permission to have an autopsy performed. The pathologist reported severe diffuse atherosclerosis of all three coronary arteries with poor collateral circulation. The pathologist also found evidence of an old inferior wall infarct but attributed death to total occlusion of the main stem of the left coronary artery. The blood supply to the anterior and some of the posterior myocardium was completely cut off, resulting in a massive, lethal infarction of the left ventricle, which also caused the arrhythmias that preceded death. Nothing would have restored Jim's health — his disease was too advanced.

Could we have done anything more for Jim? Usually, a patient this young would have been taken to the cardiac cathcterization laboratory for a coronary visualization, once an acute MI was ruled out. The purpose is to determine whether immediate heart surgery could prevent an infarct by improving myocardial blood sup-

ply. But Jim had refused to undergo cardiac catheterization.

In contrast to this dramatic example, when heart block occurs in an older person, the symptoms may develop gradually. Because many older persons experience occasional episodes of dizziness, they blame old age or high blood pressure, and do not seek cardiac evaluation.

Before the advent of pacemakers, treatment of patients with advanced heart block was limited to providing custodial care. With no effective means for increasing cardiac output and thus increasing the oxygen supply to the brain, we were helpless to prevent progressive mental deterioration. Certainly, we've come a long way in cardiac treatment since then.

SKILLCHECK 6

Whenever examining a tracing for a possible AV block, you'll want to closely examine the length of the P-R interval, the relationship of P waves to QRS complexes, and, in second degree blocks, the R-R interval. Paying particular attention to those EKG segments, see if you can correctly analyze the following strips.

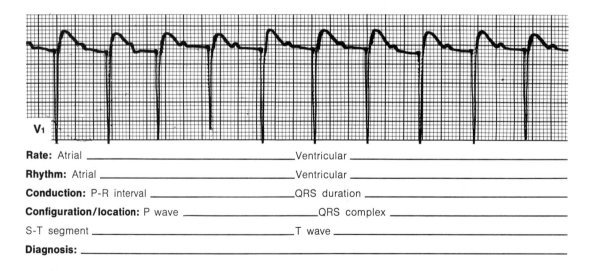

Rate: Atrial _____ Ventricular _____

Rhythm: Atrial _____ Ventricular _____

Conduction: P-R interval _____ QRS duration _____

Configuration/location: P wave _____ QRS complex _____

S-T segment _____ T wave _____

Diagnosis: _____

II

Rate: Atrial _____ Ventricular _____

Rhythm: Atrial _____ Ventricular _____

Conduction: P-R interval _____ QRS duration _____

Configuration/location: P wave _____ QRS complex _____

S-T segment _____ T wave _____

Diagnosis: _____

V₁

Rate: Atrial _____ Ventricular _____

Rhythm: Atrial _____ Ventricular _____

Conduction: P-R interval _____ QRS duration _____

Configuration/location: P wave _____ QRS complex _____

S-T segment _____ T wave _____

Diagnosis: _____

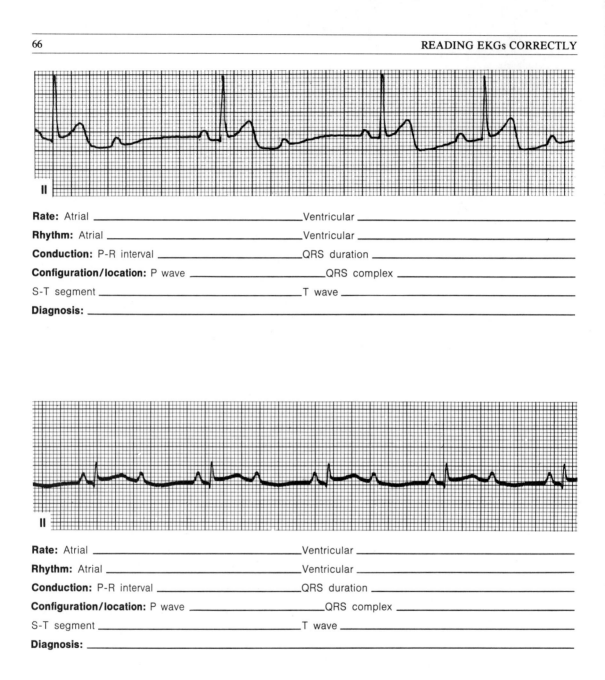

Rate: Atrial _____ Ventricular _____

Rhythm: Atrial _____ Ventricular _____

Conduction: P-R interval _____ QRS duration _____

Configuration/location: P wave _____ QRS complex _____

S-T segment _____ T wave _____

Diagnosis: _____

Rate: Atrial _____ Ventricular _____

Rhythm: Atrial _____ Ventricular _____

Conduction: P-R interval _____ QRS duration _____

Configuration/location: P wave _____ QRS complex _____

S-T segment _____ T wave _____

Diagnosis: _____

7 Ventricular arrhythmias: Possible exceptions

In the preceding chapters, we've stressed the importance of considering your patient's whole picture — his history, clinical observations, laboratory data, and so forth — before judging the seriousness of the arrhythmia and determining what treatment, if any, might be required. But with ventricular arrhythmias, discussed in this chapter, the EKG is the best means of diagnosing the arrhythmia and determining its seriousness.

Ventricular arrhythmias are almost always serious. Usually they occur suddenly and are often rapidly fatal despite vigorous treatment. On the other hand, like arrhythmias discussed earlier, they are occasionally benign, as the following case illustrates.

Harold S., a 29-year-old pharmaceutical representative, requested a physical examination required for renewal of his amateur pilot's license. Much to his and the doctor's surprise, Harold's EKG showed definite signs of ectopic ventricular activity (PVCs). Consequently, the family doctor referred him to a cardiologist, who

admitted him to our CCU for evaluation.

Despite the low incidence of myocardial infarction in men under 30, we considered this a possibility but quickly ruled it out based on Harold's history, laboratory data, EKG, and physical examination.

Continuous cardiac monitoring showed that Harold did indeed have frequent episodes of ventricular ectopic activity — i.e., PVCs followed by short runs of ventricular tachycardia (Figure 1). When we saw the tachycardia on the monitor, we'd run to Harold's room only to find him resting quietly or even asleep. When awake he felt no ill effects from the disturbance. Yet he was aware of it; he'd stop in the middle of a conversation to tell us, "It's happening again," then go on speaking as though everything were normal.

We treated him with various drugs — lidocaine, quinidine, and procainamide — but none of them had any effect on the arrhythmia. After several days of observation but still no success with drug therapy, Harold underwent

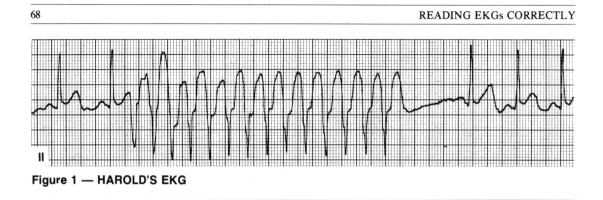

Figure 1 — HAROLD'S EKG

cardiac catheterization for a suspected cardio-myopathy. But his coronary angiography and the rest of his catheterization data showed no cardiac damage. An exercise tolerance test showed that during exercise his PVCs disappeared as did the ventricular tachycardia.

Eventually we discharged Harold on propranolol, 10 mg t.i.d., which partially controlled the ventricular tachycardia. He still flies his own plane and appears to be living a full and normal life without any serious effects from his arrhythmia.

But admittedly, Harold is unusual. Why didn't he have any ill effects from an arrhythmia that in most patients would be considered ominous? As with the arrhythmias discussed earlier, the answer lies in the effect on cardiac output. Harold had good peripheral perfusion despite his PVCs and tachycardia. Even as the PVCs appeared on his monitor, his pulse became only slightly weaker. Had we been unable to feel the pulse when we saw a PVC, we'd have known that the ventricular contractions were unable to maintain good cardiac output.

Varieties of PVCs
PVCs *may* occur in seemingly healthy persons like Harold. They are more common, though, when the heart is diseased or injured. They occur rarely in a child or infant, commonly in a 50-year-old cardiac patient, almost invariably in a 70-year-old.

PVCs originate in an ectopic focus of the ventricular myocardium. On the EKG, a PVC appears as a wide, bizarre-shaped QRS complex with no preceding P wave. Often the QRS points in the opposite direction from the patient's normal QRS complexes. The T wave that follows also is wider and larger and usually points in the opposite direction from the QRS complex (see Figures 2A and 2B).

What happens is that the ventricles are stimulated prematurely (right after their repolarization phase) and contract before the expected time.

The ventricular depolarization-repolarization cycle consists of five periods: the normal excitable period, the absolute refractory period, the relative refractory period, the vulnerable period, and the supernormal period.

The cycle begins (the normal excitable period) when the impulse reaches the bundle of His, causing ventricular depolarization to begin and ventricular contraction to take place.

After the contraction, a short period of relaxation occurs, in which the ventricles are resting, or repolarizing. The earliest stage of repolarization is the second phase, or absolute refractory period. During this phase, the cardiac cells are depleted of energy so they can't respond to any stimuli. On the EKG, this period begins during the QRS complex and lasts into the S-T segment.

During the third or relative refractory period,

the cells can respond only to strong stimuli. This period extends from the remainder of the S-T segment to the early part of the T wave.

The vulnerable period — the fourth phase — is the most delicate in the cycle. Some of the cells are fully repolarized, others partially repolarized. On the EKG the vulnerable period occurs at the peak of the T wave. In any patient, particularly one who has organic heart disease, a single PVC occurring during this phase (R on T phenomenon) could initiate ventricular tachycardia or ventricular fibrillation.

Thus, the seriousness of PVCs is determined not only by how often they occur, but also by how close they are to the T wave of the preceding beat (coupling interval).

The fifth phase of the cycle, or supernormal period, occurs when repolarization is nearly completed; hence, the ventricles can respond to stimulation. This is when most PVCs occur. On the EKG, the supernormal period is at the end of the T wave.

If you suspect that the patient is having PVCs, check his rhythm strip for two things. First, see if each PVC occurs at exactly the same time after a normal beat. To do this, measure from the normal QRS complex to the PVC, and then check this interval for all the other premature beats. If all intervals are exactly the same, *fixed coupling* is occurring, i.e., the interval between the normal and abnormal beats has not varied. To be sure coupling remains fixed, be alert to any changes in the interval.

Second, observe the pause after the PVC. Measure three consecutive QRS complexes. Then compare this interval with the interval occupied by the PVC and its preceding and succeeding QRS complexes. If the intervals are the same, or nearly so, the PVC has produced a *compensatory pause;* i.e., enough time was allowed after the PVC for the SA node to reset itself and resume normal conduction.

If the pause is less than compensatory, you

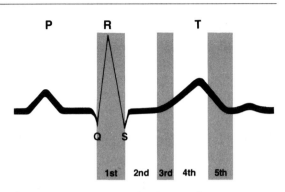

Depolarization-repolarization cycle
The ventricular depolarization-repolarization cycle consists of five periods: (1) the normal excitable period, (2) the absolute refractory period, (3) the relative refractory period, (4) the vulnerable period, and (5) the supernormal period.

should suspect that the premature beat is not a PVC but a premature atrial contraction (PAC) or a junctional premature beat. The QRS complexes of these arrhythmias may resemble those of PVCs on the rhythm strip, but they generally don't have fixed coupling. If the diagnosis is in doubt, suspect the worst and treat the patient for PVCs.

PVCs may be *unifocal* or *multifocal.* All unifocal PVCs look alike because they originate in the same single ectopic focus (Figure 2A). Multifocal PVCs, on the other hand, do not look alike — they change configuration and direction — because they originate from more than one irritable ectopic focus (Figure 2B). Multifocal PVCs, often a sign of digitalis toxicity or severe myocardial disease, are more dangerous than unifocal PVCs.

Sometimes (although not commonly) a PVC will occur between two normal cycles. Called *interpolated PVCs,* they do not disturb the heart's basic sinus rhythm.

The most benign type of PVC is probably the *fusion beat,* which stimulates the ventricles at the same time that the normal stimulus occurs. Thus, on the rhythm strip, the QRS complex is wide, but it occurs at the expected time without a compensatory pause.

Still another type of PVC, usually seen only in ICU patients, is *parasystole* or pararhythm. In this arrhythmia, the patient's own basic rhythm and a parasystole are functioning independently. The parasystolic focus discharges a regular stimulus, causing PVCs at any time in the cycle — as fusion beats, interpolated beats, and other random beats. Although the parasystole is perfectly regular, the coupling time *varies* with each PVC; therefore, a parasystole could occur during the vulnerable period, but rarely causes a run of ventricular tachycardia.

How PVCs are treated

Although isolated PVCs may require no treatment, those occurring in clusters or salvos (groups of two, three, or five) do require treatment. So do frequent PVCs (more than five or six per minute).

The chief aim of treatment is to quiet the irritable myocardium, best accomplished by administering a lidocaine bolus, followed by a continuous drip. But what if lidocaine is contraindicated, as in severe AV block or allergy? Often, procainamide will do just as well. Or, quinidine may be given by mouth. Some physicians prefer a combination of drugs. Or in some cases, the only thing required is good respiratory care (relieving hypoxia) or adding KCl to an I.V.

PVCs tend to occur in patients with slow heart rates; hence, PVCs are often associated with poor cardiac output. Restoring adequate output can best be accomplished by inserting a temporary pacemaker if severe bradycardia or AV block are present.

A variety of measures may be used in a single case, as the following shows.

Michael C., age 45, was admitted to our CCU complaining of substernal pain. His EKG showed changes in leads V_1 and V_6 on his EKG. His S-T segment was elevated indicating a possible anterolateral myocardial infarction. He had a normal sinus rhythm with rare PVCs.

Two hours later, the PVCs were occurring at a rate of five to six per minute, all unifocal. Our standing orders called for administering a bolus of lidocaine, 50 mg. If the PVCs were occurring at a rate greater than five per minute, we were to start a piggyback drip of lidocaine, 2 Gm in 500 cc of 5% dextrose in water (producing a concentration of 4 mg per cc, which we controlled by microdrip).

It became obvious that the lidocaine alone wasn't going to stop Michael's PVCs — besides he would get too much I.V. fluid if we continued to use only lidocaine — so we added quinidine, 200 mg q.i.d., by mouth. The combination

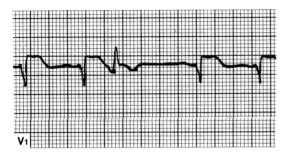

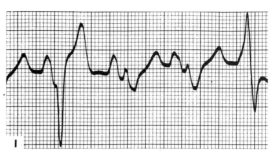

Figure 2A — UNIFOCAL PVCs

EKG Criteria:

1. QRS complex wide, bizarre, distorted and usually deflects in opposite direction from patient's
   normal QRS.
2. T wave of PVC deflects in opposite direction from
   QRS complex.
3. P waves are not usually visible.
4. Compensatory pause follows PVC.

Figure 2B — MULTIFOCAL PVCs

Treatment

Administer or apply alone or in combination:

- Lidocaine, 50-100 mg, I.V., as a bolus followed by
  an I.V. of 2 Gm lidocaine in 500 cc 5% glucose in
  water to be infused at a rate of 1-4 mg/min.
- Procainamide (Pronestyl) I.V., 1 Gm, in 500 cc 5%
  glucose in water plus oral dosages of 250-500 mg
  if tolerated.
- Potassium chloride I.V.
- Quinidine by mouth.
- Temporary pacemaker.

If PVC induced by digitalis, withhold dosage; if
induced by hypoxia, give oxygen.

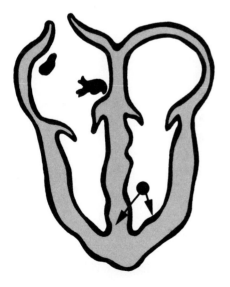

Pathway for ventricular arrhythmias

*Impulses for ventricular arrhythmias bypass the
atria altogether; instead, they come directly
from single or multiple ectopic foci in the
ventricles.*

Ventricular tachycardia often is precipitated by a PVC during the ventricular repolarization cycle.

quieted the ventricular irritability. After 3 hours of no further PVCs, we discontinued the lidocaine only to have the PVCs start again — this time in pairs (Figure 3).

Because paired PVCs pose an increased danger of ventricular tachycardia, we decided to quickly substitute procainamide by I.V. piggyback, 1 Gm in 500 cc of 5% dextrose in water, plus 250 mg by mouth q3h. We stopped the quinidine.

After 2 days of procainamide therapy, we discontinued the I.V. and maintained Michael on oral procainamide. He had no more PVCs, and the rest of his hospitalization was uneventful.

Whatever the treatment, your responsibilities in caring for patients with PVCs are as follows:

1. Decide whether the PVCs are unifocal or multifocal.

2. Check the location of the PVCs in respect to the T waves on the rhythm strip.

3. Observe the effects of the PVCs on the patient.

4. Be alert for runs of three or more PVCs (ventricular tachycardia).

5. Note what medications the patient has been taking, particularly those that might cause PVCs.

6. Know *when* to call the doctor and *what* to report.

7. Be certain that medication and equipment are ready for any treatment that may be needed.

8. Thus prepared, remain calm and confident in any eventuality.

Ventricular tachycardia

In many instances ventricular tachycardia is precipitated by a PVC that occurs in the vulnerable period of the ventricular repolarization cycle (the R on T phenomenon). In normal patients, the ventricular rate is 20 to 40 beats per minute; in ventricular tachycardia, the rate ranges from 50 (slow ventricular tachycardia) to 220 (rapid ventricular tachycardia). On the

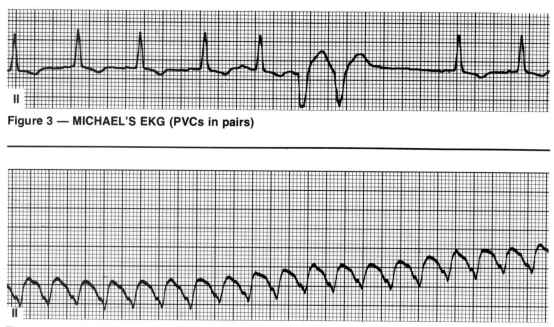

Figure 3 — MICHAEL'S EKG (PVCs in pairs)

Figure 4 — VENTRICULAR TACHYCARDIA

EKG Criteria:
1. Ventricular rate ranges from 50 to 220 per minute.
2. QRS is wide and bizarre.
3. R-R intervals usually are regular but a slight irregularity may occur.
4. P waves are obscured by QRS complex.

Note: A group of three PVCs constitutes a short run of ventricular tachycardia.

Treatment
Administer or apply alone or in combination:
• Lidocaine (Xylocaine)
• Procainamide (Pronestyl)
• Quinidine
Insert temporary pacemaker for slow rates with short runs of ventricular tachycardia.
Apply direct-current shock if patient is rapidly deteriorating.

EKG, ventricular tachycardia can be identified by wide but uniform QRS complexes and a regular rhythm (see Figure 4).

Since most patients can't tolerate high ventricular rates for long, they must be treated. For short runs of tachycardia (five to six beats alternating with slow regular rhythm), lidocaine may suffice, but for longer runs, a direct-current shock of 250 to 400 w/sec is usually necessary. This should be followed with administration of myocardial suppressant drugs (e.g., lidocaine or procainamide) or a precordial thump.

Ventricular flutter
Sometimes called "fine ventricular fibrillation," ventricular flutter often appears as a transient state between ventricular tachycardia and ventricular fibrillation. In fact, it may be so transient that it sweeps the monitor screen before you can recognize it. On the rhythm strip, it appears as a

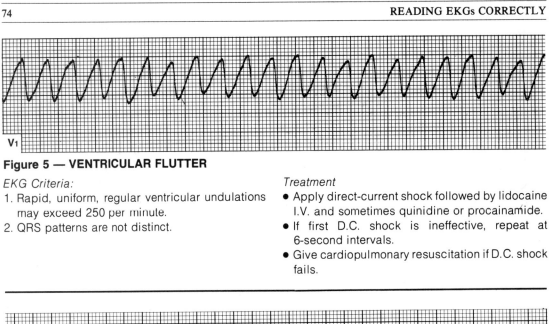

Figure 5 — VENTRICULAR FLUTTER

EKG Criteria:

1. Rapid, uniform, regular ventricular undulations may exceed 250 per minute.
2. QRS patterns are not distinct.

Treatment

• Apply direct-current shock followed by lidocaine I.V. and sometimes quinidine or procainamide.
• If first D.C. shock is ineffective, repeat at 6-second intervals.
• Give cardiopulmonary resuscitation if D.C. shock fails.

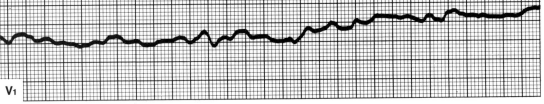

Figure 6 — VENTRICULAR FIBRILLATION

EKG Criterion:

1. Rapid, chaotic, ventricular rhythm lacks pattern.

Treatment

• Administer immediate direct-current shock of 400 w/sec followed by I.V. lidocaine or pronestyl and cardiopulmonary resuscitation.

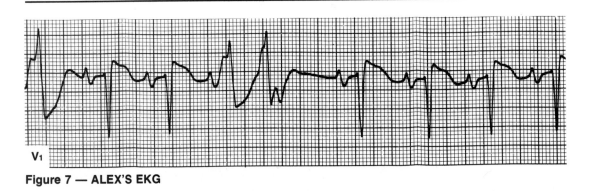

Figure 7 — ALEX'S EKG

clearly defined series of configurations that resemble the letter "m" (Figure 5). Clinically, the patient with ventricular flutter will show signs of poor cardiac output. He may appear dead, may have a mild convulsive seizure, and may be incontinent.

If you're at a patient's bedside when he develops ventricular flutter, you might try a precordial thump with your closed fist. Usually, though, he'll need a direct-current shock of 400 w/sec immediately. Until the defibrillator arrives, be sure to maintain his airway and circulation by mouth-to-mouth breathing and chest decompression.

Ventricular fibrillation

Once you've seen this arrhythmia, you'll never forget it. Ventricular fibrillation appears on the monitor as an uncoordinated, unrhythmic tracing with no pattern that resembles any arrhythmia we've presented so far. The rhythm strip shown in Figure 6 is an example. The patient may appear dead, with incontinence, a complete loss of sensorium, and possible tremors or seizures.

You must call for help immediately and begin treatment. The only effective treatment is direct-current shock of 400 to 500 w/sec. One shock seldom is enough; if the first shock doesn't immediately reverse the arrhythmia, deliver another within 6 seconds. Keep delivering shocks — five times, if necessary. If shock is ineffective, CPR should be initiated as soon as help arrives. I.V. NaHCO₃ should be started and, if possible, samples obtained for blood gas determination. Also, the patient must be intubated with an endotracheal tube and ventilated.

One person should prepare the medications the doctor may need — bicarbonate, vasopressors, lidocaine, epinephrine, and calcium gluconate. Have several intracardiac needles and syringes also ready.

Sometimes it's possible to reverse ventricular fibrillation with a precordial thump, direct-current shock, and drugs; sometimes it's not. On our unit, we've also tried intracardiac pacing on occasion, but we can't claim success with this treatment.

Guarded prognosis

While success in reversing ventricular fibrillation partly depends on how promptly you recognize the arrhythmia and act, it depends heavily on one factor you can't control: the condition of the patient's myocardium. Indeed, any ventricular arrhythmia in a patient with a severely damaged myocardium implies a grave prognosis, as in the following case.

Alex, age 62, had had two previous infarctions before admission to our CCU. The initial diagnosis, possible lateral wall infarction, was based on a complaint of severe angina and an EKG that showed changes in the S-T segment in leads V_5 and V_6.

Alex's admission EKG showed a moderately fast heart rate of 110, with occasional PVCs (less than five per minute). Following standing orders for PVCs, we administered lidocaine drip, 4 mg per cc (2 Gm lidocaine in 500 cc of 5% dextrose in water).

Soon after admission, Alex began to have more frequent PVCs (Figure 7). They were unifocal, but they came in pairs, which meant that Alex could quickly develop ventricular tachycardia and even ventricular fibrillation. We had no doubt that the ectopic beats were indeed PVCs and that they were not responding to lidocaine. So, we changed to procainamide, 1 Gm in 500 cc of 5% dextrose in water, and also administered 1 mg of propranolol by slow I.V. push. Soon the PVCs disappeared, so we stopped the procainamide drip that evening and gave it by mouth.

Later that night, the PVCs recurred in pairs. Again we administered I.V. procainamide, but with no effect. We also administered propran-

Asystole is always life-threatening but not always fatal. Many patients survive episodes of cardiac arrest, depending on the condition of their heart and on their treatment.

olol. Still no effect. Yet, we detected no sign of congestive failure; his CVP was normal and his chest was clear.

Before long, the PVCs began occurring in groups of three to five (short runs of ventricular tachycardia). Again, we tried lidocaine — again no effect. Then Alex became hypotensive — perhaps partially due to the lidocaine — and he was deteriorating clinically. Before we could insert a temporary pacemaker, he had a short run of ventricular tachycardia, which quickly progressed to ventricular fibrillation. We administered several direct-current shocks of 400 w/sec, but failed to resuscitate him.

As a last resort, we inserted a transthoracic needle into the ventricle and threaded a pacemaker electrode into the heart. This too failed. Alex's myocardium was just too badly damaged from his previous infarctions.

Asystole

Of all cardiac emergencies, asystole (cardiac arrest or ventricular standstill) strikes the most fear in nurses. And little wonder. It is always life-threatening. But that doesn't mean that it's always fatal. In fact, many patients, particularly young ones with no serious underlying medical problems, survive episodes of cardiac arrest. Whether they do depends on the condition of their heart muscles, function of the pulmonary system, and the alertness and informed action of nurses and doctors.

Literally translated, asystole means absence of contraction — the heart doesn't beat. So, it typically appears on a monitor as a straight line. But that isn't always the case: asystole also can appear as a chaotic imprint (Figure 8) showing some excitability of myocardium, which indicates end stage ventricular fibrillation.

A common cause of asystole is hypoxia from impaired respiratory function. It also can arise from several other noncardiac problems — to name a few, respiratory impairment caused by

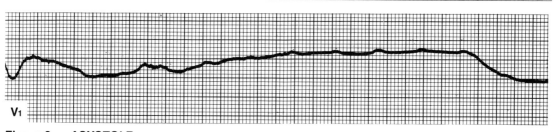

V_1

Figure 8 — ASYSTOLE

EKG Criteria:
1. Either a straight line EKG or some chaotic in-comprehensible imprint.

Treatment
- Sharp precordial thump
- CPR (immediate)
- Defibrillate with 400 w/sec.
- Drugs:
  $NaHCO_3$ I.V.
  Intracardiac epinephrine
  Calcium gluconate I.V.
  Vasopressors (Levophed, Aramine)
- Transthoracic pacemaker
- Intra-aortic balloon pump

anesthesia, drug overdosage, hemorrhage, or anaphylactic reactions. If it occurs in a cardiac patient who is being constantly monitored, it usually does so at the end stage of resuscitation or is preceded by marked, uncontrolled episodes of ventricular irritability.

Asystole is a true emergency. When it occurs, you must act quickly to initiate cardiopulmonary resuscitation. Start I.V. sodium bicarbonate and prepare an intracardiac injection of epinephrine for the doctor to administer when he arrives. In extreme cases the doctor may even shock the patient with 400 w/sec or insert an intracardiac pacemaker electrode through the anterior chest wall.

Bundle branch block

Conduction delays or blocks can occur in the bundle branches for the same reasons that they occur in the AV node or bundle of His. Although bundle branch blocks occasionally occur in healthy persons, they occur more commonly in patients with coronary artery disease or hypertension. Treatment is directed toward the associated heart disease rather than toward the block itself.

There are actually three bundle branches, because the left bundle branch divides into an anterior-superior division and a posterior-inferior division. The right bundle branch, however, is long and slender and doesn't divide until it reaches the endocardial surface of the right ventricle near the septum.

EKG changes of bundle branch block are best seen in the precordial leads V_1 through V_6. Lead V_1 is the one we use to make the distinction between left and right bundle branch block, although with experience you will detect changes in the other leads as well.

Lead V_1 normally consists of a deep S wave

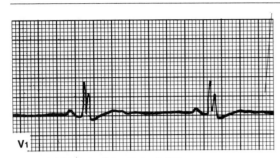

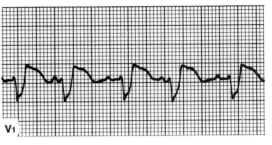

9A — RIGHT BUNDLE BLOCK

EKG Criteria:

1. QRS prolonged to 0.12 seconds or more and is entirely above the isoelectric line in lead V₁.
2. Right precordial lead (e.g. V₁₋₂) shows rSR′complex with S-T depression and inverted T waves.

Treatment
- None may be needed.
- Treat underlying heart disease.

9B — LEFT BUNDLE BLOCK

EKG Criteria

1. QRS prolonged to 0.12 seconds or more and is below the isoelectric line in lead V₁.
2. Deep S wave appears in V₁.

Treatment
- None may be needed.
- Treat underlying heart disease.

---

preceded by a small R wave. In right bundle branch block (Figure 9A) the R wave broadens or slurs and the QRS, which is now called rSR′, looks like an "M." Also, in right bundle branch block, the QRS is above the isoelectric line (a positive deflection).

In left bundle branch block (Figure 9B) the S wave deepens and most of the QRS complex is below the isoelectric line (a negative deflection). In both left and right bundle branch block the QRS duration is 0.12 seconds or more.

That the QRS complex is prolonged is readily understandable when we consider the mechanism of bundle branch block. Usually these blocks occur near the origin of the branch involved. When the impulse reaches the blocked area, it cannot continue; it must find an alternate route to complete ventricular depolarization, or its conduction through the blocked area is delayed.

In right bundle branch block, conduction is normal through the left bundle branch and left ventricle. Because of the blocked right bundle branch, the right ventricle can be stimulated only by an impulse transmitted to it by way of the left ventricle. Conversely, in left bundle branch block, conduction is normal through the right bundle branch, so the left ventricle is stimulated by an impulse from the right ventricle.

Such detours cause delays in transmission of the impulse, which is reflected by a widening of the QRS complex. This widened QRS is the clue to bundle branch blocks.

A subclassification of complete bundle branch blocks, which we've been describing, is incomplete bundle branch block. Incomplete BBB, which is more common than complete BBB, shows all the abnormalities of a bundle branch block except that the QRS interval is 0.10 to 0.11 seconds. Usually it occurs where a congenital defect or ventricular strain is present, such as with cor pulmonale and ventricular hypertrophy.

SKILLCHECK 7

Generally speaking, the clue to ventricular arrhythmias and bundle branch blocks rests with the QRS. In ventricular arrhythmias, the QRS may be inverted, indistinct, or bizarre. In bundle branch blocks, the QRS is prolonged and rises above or falls below the isoelectric line. As you analyze the following EKGs, note the variations in the QRS complexes.

V₁

Rate: Atrial _____ Ventricular _____

Rhythm: Atrial _____ Ventricular _____

Conduction: P-R interval _____ QRS duration _____

Configuration/location: P wave _____ QRS complex _____

S-T segment _____ T wave _____

Diagnosis: _____

V₁

Rate: Atrial _____ Ventricular _____

Rhythm: Atrial _____ Ventricular _____

Conduction: P-R interval _____ QRS duration _____

Configuration/location: P wave _____ QRS complex _____

S-T segment _____ T wave _____

Diagnosis: _____

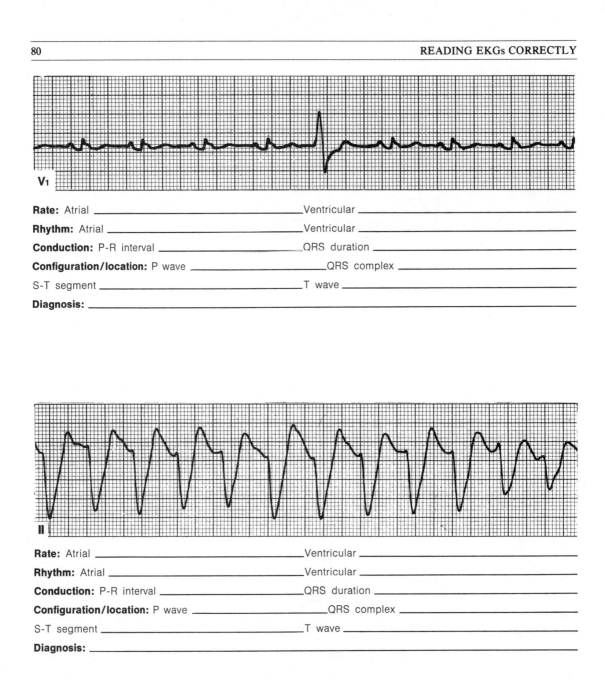

Rate: Atrial _____Ventricular _____

Rhythm: Atrial _____Ventricular _____

Conduction: P-R interval _____QRS duration _____

Configuration/location: P wave _____QRS complex _____

S-T segment _____T wave _____

Diagnosis: _____

Rate: Atrial _____Ventricular _____

Rhythm: Atrial _____Ventricular _____

Conduction: P-R interval _____QRS duration _____

Configuration/location: P wave _____QRS complex _____

S-T segment _____T wave _____

Diagnosis: _____

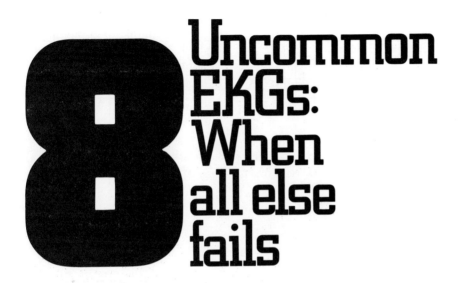

8 Uncommon EKGs: When all else fails

In the past five chapters, we've presented the arrhythmias you're most likely to see in your everyday practice. If you become thoroughly familiar with them, you'll be able to accurately interpret almost every EKG you may encounter. Still, others do exist. Even though they are highly uncommon, you should be aware of their names, salient features, and usual treatment.

The following sample strips, accompanied by capsule information, should give you an adequate briefing on these uncommon arrhythmias. Check a tracing for these *only* when you have exhausted all other possibilities from the preceding chapters.

SA block
SA block is any block that prevents an impulse from the SA node from reaching the atria. Because of the interference with impulse transmission, there are no atrial or ventricular contractions. So, a cardiac cycle is missing on the EKG.

Rhythm remains normal, though. That is, if you measure the tracing you'll find that the distance between QRS complexes before and after the dropped beat is *exactly* twice as long as normal. (This feature distinguishes SA block from sinus arrest.)

SA block can be caused by excess digitalis or quinidine, vagal stimulation (e.g., carotid massage), or organic heart disease in the area of the SA node.

Blocked PAC
A blocked PAC is a premature impulse arising from an atrial ectopic focus that doesn't reach the ventricles. Cardiologists theorize that the PACs aren't conducted because of the refractoriness of the AV node.

In a blocked PAC, a P wave (often abnormal in configuration) occurs without a QRS following it, much like SA block. Unlike SA block, though, the rhythm is disturbed; the interval between QRS complexes is *longer or shorter*

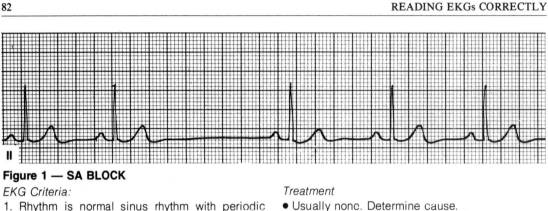

Figure 1 — SA BLOCK

EKG Criteria:

1. Rhythm is normal sinus rhythm with periodic pauses where an entire cardiac cycle (P, QRS, T) is dropped.
2. The dropped cycle doesn't interfere with the normal rhythm; the interval of the dropped beat equals a normal cycle.

Treatment

• Usually none. Determine cause.

than two normal QRS intervals.

Wolff Parkinson White (WPW)

WPW, or accelerated conduction, most frequently occurs in men under 30. In it, impulses from the SA node can penetrate the AV node in the usual fashion or they can bypass the AV node and reach the ventricles early, resulting in a short or absent P-R interval.

Because of the accelerated conduction, patients in WPW are prone to rapid heart rates. You should suspect WPW in any patient with frequent bouts of paroxysmal tachycardia with QRS complexes that look like bundle branch blocks. Figure 3, showing a classical example of WPW, illustrates the *WPW syndrome*. In *true WPW,* however, the EKG would also show runs of paroxysmal supraventricular tachycardia.

AV dissociation

When the atria and ventricles are controlled by two different pacemakers due to impaired conduction through the AV node, the condition is

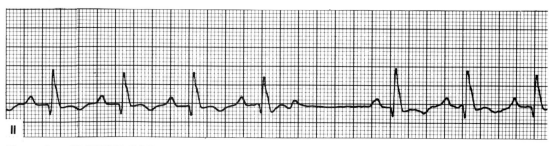

II

Figure 2 — BLOCKED PAC

EKG Criteria:

1. P wave occurs early and is often of a different configuration and direction than normal P wave.
2. No QRS complex follows premature P wave.
3. Interval with dropped QRS is less than a normal cycle.

Treatment

- If numerous blocked PACs occur, consider hypokalemia and check for digitalis intoxication or ischemia.

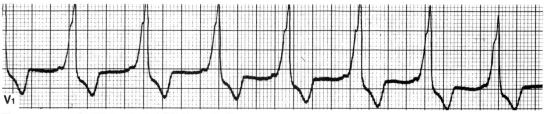

V₁

Figure 3 — WOLFF PARKINSON WHITE (WPW)

EKG Criteria:

1. P-R interval is very short (less than 0.10 sec).
2. QRS complex is wide (0.11-0.14 sec) or slurred (looks like bundle branch block).
3. Delta waves, which occur at upstroke of QRS complex, are present.
4. Tracing shows runs of paroxysmal tachycardia, which appear as ventricular tachycardia.

Treatment

- Quinidine sometimes effective.
- Pronestyl sometimes effective.
- Bedrest for tachycardia.
- Ligation of AV node and permanent bipolar pacemaker.

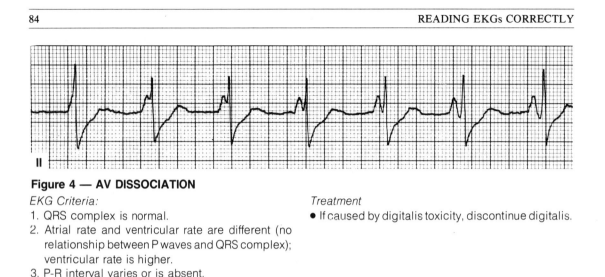

II

Figure 4 — AV DISSOCIATION

EKG Criteria:
1. QRS complex is normal.
2. Atrial rate and ventricular rate are different (no relationship between P waves and QRS complex); ventricular rate is higher.
3. P-R interval varies or is absent.

Treatment
● If caused by digitalis toxicity, discontinue digitalis.

known as AV dissociation. In this condition, the SA node paces the atria and the AV node paces the ventricles. The ventricular rate therefore is higher than the atrial rate, causing junctional tachycardia. AV dissociation is often caused by digitalis toxicity. In almost every case, it is a transient arrhythmia.

On an EKG, AV dissociation produces a normal QRS complex but varying atrial and ventricular rates. Because the P waves are unrelated to the QRS complexes, the P-R intervals will vary or may even be absent.

9 Insight into two life-threatening conditions

An EKG can be invaluable in diagnosing arrhythmias. But it also can be invaluable in diagnosing several conditions that can precipitate arrhythmias — specifically, congenital heart disease, pericarditis, pericardial effusion, electrolyte imbalance, and myocardial infarction.

Unless you work in a CCU, you'll probably never see the first three of those conditions. But no matter where you work, you're apt to see electrolyte imbalance and myocardial infarction. That's why your understanding of the EKG changes that these conditions produce can be so important.

True, the EKG won't always be your first warning of these conditions. In some cases, you may discover them through other means — through lab tests for electrolyte imbalance or through simple observation and the patient's medical history for myocardial infarction or electrolyte imbalance. But often EKG changes can be your first clue to these dangerous conditions, *if* you know what to look for.

Detecting potassium imbalances

Both calcium and potassium play an important role in cardiac rhythm. For the most part, though, EKG interpretation has only limited value in detecting calcium imbalances since the EKG changes are almost imperceptible: a slightly shortened Q-T segment in hypercalcemia and a lengthened S-T segment in hypocalcemia.

But with potassium imbalance, the EKG changes can be a useful diagnostic tool.

Potassium imbalance affects the electrical activity of muscle, including the myocardium. At a normal blood level of 3.5 to 5.0 mEq/L, potassium helps keep the heart in normal rhythm. But an excess or deficit of potassium can cause dangerous arrhythmias.

If mild, *hypokalemia* (low blood potassium levels) may cause only muscular weakness and fatigue. The myocardial effects include atrial or ventricular irritability. But if severe, it can cause severe muscle weakness, paralysis, atrial

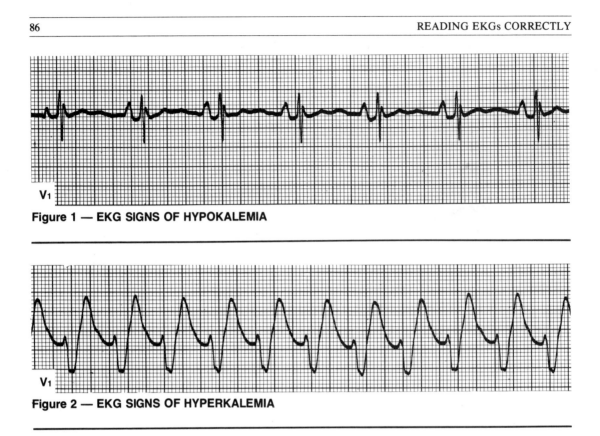

Figure 1 — EKG SIGNS OF HYPOKALEMIA

Figure 2 — EKG SIGNS OF HYPERKALEMIA

tachycardia with varying degrees of block, and ventricular premature beats that may progress to ventricular tachycardia and fibrillation. These dangerous arrhythmias are particularly apt to occur in patients on diuretics, which can cause potassium depletion. With hypokalemia, digitalis toxicity can readily occur.

Early signs of hypokalemia are prominent U waves, a prolonged Q-U interval, and flat or inverted T waves (Figure 1). Usually the T waves will not flatten or invert until potassium depletion reaches a severe stage.

Though less common, severe *hyperkalemia* (high potassium blood level) also can be highly dangerous since it can prevent the heart from conducting its electrical impulses. This can cause paroxysmal tachycardia, premature contractions, atrial flutter, atrial fibrillation, or cardiac arrest. Cardiac arrest is usually preceded by loss of P waves, widened QRS complexes, and eventually ventricular tachycardia, ventricular fibrillation, or standstill.

Early signs of hyperkalemia are small P waves, a widened QRS, and especially tall, tent-shaped T waves (Figure 2). These changes relate almost precisely to specific potassium blood levels: usually changes in the T waves indicate a level of 6.0 to 7.0 mEq/L and widening of the QRS indicates a level of 8.0 to 9.0 mEq/L (a level that can quickly result in cardiac death).

EKGs and MIs

Unfortunately, EKGs won't always help you recognize myocardial infarction. Many infarction patients never develop an arrhythmia, since the infarcted area may not interfere with the depolarization-repolarization cycle or with cardiac conduction to any great extent. Some may not develop any EKG changes for several days, when they begin to show up on serial tracings. And others with an abnormally shaped chest or an abnormally positioned heart may never show characteristic EKG changes indicating an acute MI. Sometimes, too, the EKG changes may be so transient that you'll miss them on routine tracings. Or the EKG may not detect an infarct if it's small. In such cases, you'll have to rely solely on your observations of the patient and your knowledge of his medical history and his physical exam.

But with many MI patients, the EKG can be a valuable supplement to your observations.

The most common cause of acute myocardial infarction is occlusion of a coronary artery, interfering with coronary blood flow to the myocardium. To visualize how obstruction of the blood flow can cause tissue damage and EKG changes, you should have some idea of the circulation to the myocardium (see Figure 3). Depending on the degree of oxygen deprivation caused by an obstruction, various tissue

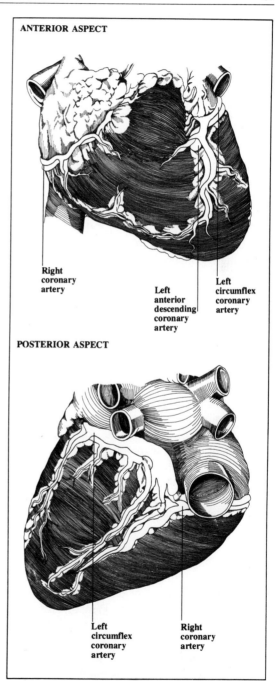

ANTERIOR ASPECT

Right coronary artery

Left anterior descending coronary artery

Left circumflex coronary artery

POSTERIOR ASPECT

Left circumflex coronary artery

Right coronary artery

Figure 3 — CIRCULATION TO MYOCARDIUM

changes can result: an inner zone of tissue necrosis (the true infarct), a surrounding zone of severe ischemia, and an outer zone of ischemia (Figure 4). The EKG changes that occur in the lead facing the damaged area depend on the stage of development (evolution) of the myocardial infarction.

The first EKG change is an elevation in the S-T segment, indicating the formation of an ischemic zone. This is called a "current of injury" pattern. Next, the T wave begins to flatten and finally inverts. Then, enlarged Q waves appear, indicating developing necrosis (true infarction). For Q waves to be "abnormal," they should be larger than one small square on the EKG paper horizontally (0.04 sec) and vertically (0.1 mv). Q waves exceeding these dimensions are "pathologic" and usually indicate areas of infarction.

Q waves may appear immediately or within the first several days after the onset of symptoms. These Q waves will remain and usually can be detected for several years after the infarction has healed.

On the other hand, elevated S-T segments will appear immediately but will return to normal within 1 to 4 weeks after the infarction. Because elevation of the S-T segment is transient, it may not appear on the first EKG if the patient delays reporting his symptoms to a physician. The T waves will become deeply and symmetrically inverted within 6 to 24 hours after the infarction and may return to normal within 2 weeks to several years later.

By coupling your knowledge about evolving EKG changes with your understanding of the leads and which areas of damage they detect, you often can determine the extent and location of cardiac damage from a patient's EKG.

Learning the leads
To assess the EKG of an MI patient, you must first assume that the patient's heart is in the normal position and that his chest is a normal shape. Then, you can localize the area of damage by picturing the areas of the heart that each EKG lead faces (i.e., the areas of electrical activity that each lead records).

The precordial leads ($V_1 — V_6$) face the anterior and lateral aspects of the heart. Consequently, they can give you the best views of damage in those areas.

Leads V_1 and V_2, on the anterior chest at the fourth intercostal space to the right and left of the sternum respectively, lie just over the anterior surface of the right ventricle. So, changes in leads V_1 or V_2 indicate damage in that area, caused by an occlusion in the right coronary artery.

Lead V_3, between the fourth and fifth intercostal spaces and to the left of the septum, lies just over the ventricular septum. It records activity of the septum and both the left and right ventricles. Changes in V_3 indicate damage in the septum or in the anterior wall of the left ventricle or right ventricle, caused by occlusion of the branches of the left anterior descending coronary artery. To decide exactly which of these areas is damaged, you'd have to examine leads V_1, V_2, and V_4 as well.

Lead V_4, placed in the fifth intercostal space, lies over the septum and anterior wall of the left ventricle. When used with V_3, V_5, or V_6, it can pinpoint left ventricular damage in either the septum or anterior wall of the left ventricle, also caused by occlusion of the branches of the left anterior descending coronary artery.

Lead V_5 faces the lateral aspect of the left ventricle, while lead V_6 faces both the lateral and slightly posterior segments of the left ventricle. Changes in V_5 and V_6 are most apt to indicate damage to the lateral wall of the left ventricle, caused by occlusion of the branches of the left circumflex coronary artery or distal left anterior descending coronary artery, although V_6 also can give you information on posterior lateral

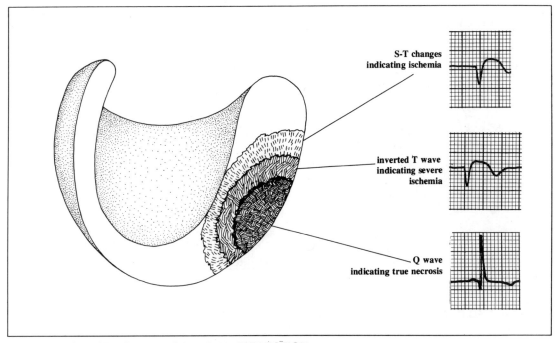

S-T changes
indicating ischemia

inverted T wave
indicating severe
ischemia

Q wave
indicating true necrosis

Figure 4 — STAGES OF A MYOCARDIAL INFARCTION

damage to the left ventricle.

Lead aVL, which views the heart from the left shoulder, also can help pinpoint damage to the lateral wall of the heart when studied with V_4, V_5, and V_6.

Of all the standard and augmented leads, aVR has the least diagnostic value. Since it faces the heart from the right shoulder, it records electrical activity in only a small portion of the right base of the heart. Except in rare cases, it isn't used for definitive diagnostic purposes.

Leads II, III, and aVF, however, record the bulk of electrical activity in the diaphragmatic (inferior) area of the heart. Therefore, EKG changes in these leads indicate inferior wall damage, usually from obstruction of the right coronary artery causing an inferior wall infarction.

In contrast, changes in leads I, aVL, and V_2-V_5 indicate damage to the anterior left ventri-

Myocardial infarction causes three changes: an inner zone of tissue necrosis, a surrounding zone of inflamed tissue, and an outer zone of ischemia.

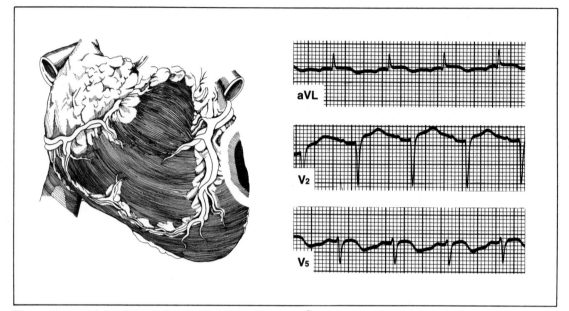

Figure 5 — EKG CHANGES WITH AN ANTERIOR INFARCTION

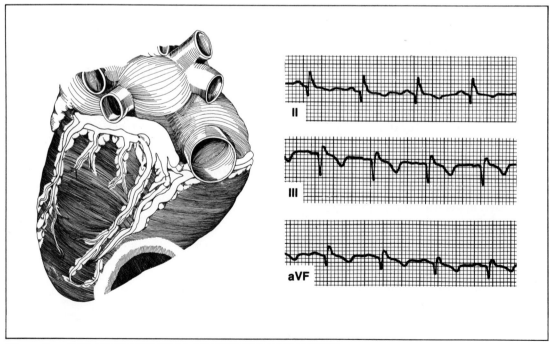

Figure 6 — EKG CHANGES WITH AN INFERIOR INFARCTION

cle (anterior wall or antero-septal infarction), caused by obstruction of the left anterior descending branch of the left coronary artery.

Finally, changes in leads I, aVL, and V4-V6 indicate lateral wall damage (lateral wall infarction) most likely caused by an obstruction of the circumflex branch of the left coronary artery. (Occasionally, though, this infarction may be caused by an obstruction of the left anterior descending coronary artery.)

Figures 5 and 6 show the specific EKG changes you'll see with two common types of infarct. Remember, though, that other conditions can produce EKG changes resembling those produced by acute myocardial infarction. For example, pericarditis, acute pulmonary embolism, myocarditis, and left ventricular hypertrophy sometimes produce similar changes. And serial changes of a relatively small myocardial infarction may be so transient that they won't be detected by a routine EKG. In these instances, your evaluation of the patient's clinical course and laboratory data will help establish the specific diagnosis.

SKILLCHECK 9

Following are a few infarct tracings. Try to assess not only the location but also the extent of myocardial damage in each one. Don't forget to pay particular attention to the lead positions.

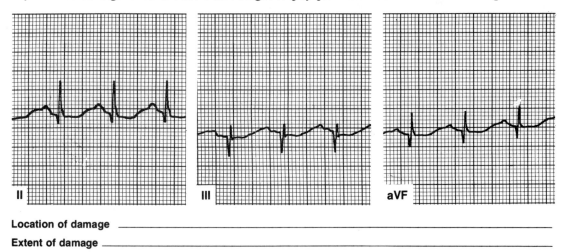

Location of damage _____

Extent of damage _____

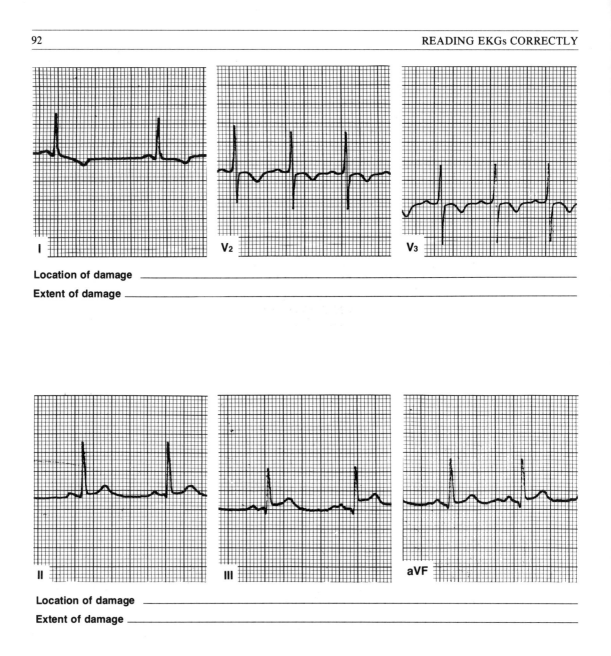

Location of damage _____

Extent of damage _____

Location of damage _____

Extent of damage _____

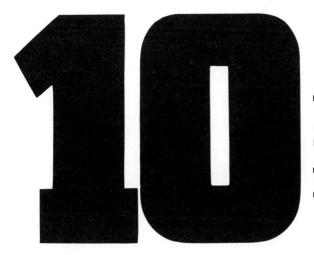

A glance at cardiac monitors

So far, we've talked about EKG tracings, those strips of paper that are a permanent record of the patient's cardiac activity. And we've repeatedly cautioned you to "measure the tracings; don't depend on your glances at the monitor."

But no discussion of EKG interpretation would be complete without some mention of cardiac monitors. Because, although they aren't the last word in EKG interpretation, they do hold a valuable place in it. Without them, all cardiac patients would be confined to bed so they could be constantly "hooked up" to a bedside electrocardiograph. And without them, you'd spend most of your time running from one patient's room to the next, trying to keep up with the tracings coming out of several electrocardiographs.

Monitors allow patients more mobility and give a quick reading on several patients at once. True, they have their limitations: greater risk of electrical interference, which can skew a reading, and the constant movement of the tracing, which doesn't allow you to measure EKG changes on the screen. But as early warning systems, monitors can be extremely useful. The trick is knowing how to operate them and how to detect mechanical errors in monitor tracings.

Components of a monitor

Although the many monitors on the market differ in design and operation, their basic components and function are quite similar.

The *oscilloscope* is the television-like screen where the patient's electrocardiogram appears. As the heart beats, the tracing moves across the oscilloscope.

The *pulse rate meter* determines the average number of cardiac cycles per minute and registers each cardiac cycle as an audible beep. (If you don't want a bedside monitor to disturb a patient, you can lower the volume of the beep with the *volume control knob*.) At the same time, a *red flasher light* blinks on every time a QRS complex appears on the oscilloscope.

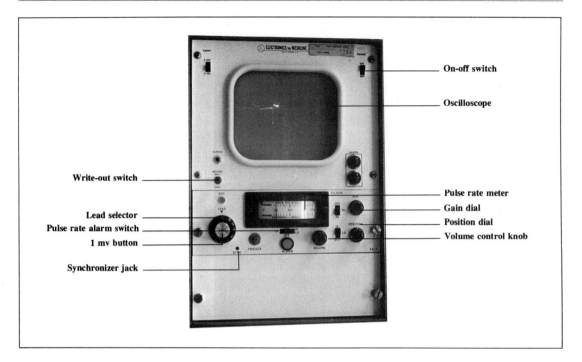

On-off switch

Oscilloscope

Pulse rate meter

Gain dial

Position dial

Volume control knob

Write-out switch

Lead selector

Pulse rate alarm switch

1 mv button

Synchronizer jack

Common monitor components

Although the many monitors on the market today differ in design, most contain the components shown here.

Connected to the pulse rate meter is a *pulse rate alarm* switch, which you can set to alert you to any abnormally high or low pulse rate. If you set the alarm system at the standard rates of 50 and 120, for example, any pulse rate falling below 50 or rising above 120 will trigger an audible alarm.

Two dials help you regulate the tracing on the oscilloscope. The *gain dial* allows you to adjust the size of the complex. And the *position dial* allows you to move the tracing up or down on the screen so you can center it or make room for other tracings (such as an arterial blood pressure reading).

If your monitor has a *lead selector,* it will allow you to choose which lead to monitor. If you notice a suspicious wave in one lead, it also will allow you to switch to another lead to double-check your suspicions. Then, if you want to measure a suspicious EKG strip, you can simply turn the *write-out switch* to the "on" position for an instantaneous write out. (If your monitor has a write-out knob with "EKG" and "Stand-by" positions, turn the knob to "EKG" for an instantaneous write-out. Turn it to "Stand-by" for an automatic write-out whenever the EKG sets off the alarm system.) Before getting a write-out, push the *1 mv button,* which will make a mark at the beginning of the strip showing the standard size of the QRS complex.

The final standard component on a monitor is the *synchronizer jack* for cardioversion. When a defibrillator is plugged into the jack, it will deliver the shock only during a QRS complex. A shock delivered at any other time would throw the patient into ventricular fibrillation. If the patient already has ventricular fibrillation, which produces no QRS complex, do not use the synchronizer jack. Instead, defibrillate rather than attempt to cardiovert the patient.

Making the connection
Since monitors are highly sensitive machines, you have to take special care in setting them up and attaching them to patients. Even some very sophisticated CCUs have no protocol for applying monitor electrodes. Yet where and how you apply them can make a big difference in the amount of information you get — or don't get — about your patient.

Before attaching the electrodes, plug in the monitor and turn it on. While it warms up, explain what you are going to do to your patient to allay his apprehension. Then select the sites for electrode placement.

We've stated that we like the conventional V_1 lead best of all the EKG leads, since it gives the most valuable information about arrhythmias. To get the best recording of this lead, we suggest you amplify it by using a modified V_1 chest lead, known as the MCL_1 (modified chest lead).

For a MCL_1, the positive electrode goes in the fourth interspace of the right sternal border, as

Monitors are highly sensitive machines; you have to take special care in setting them up and attaching them to patients.

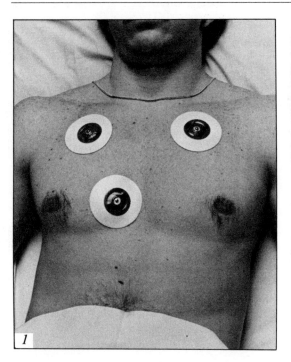

1

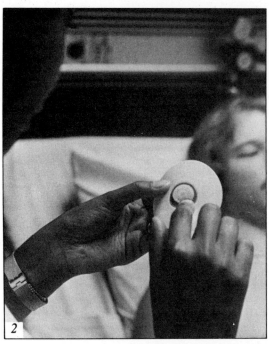

2

1. For an MCL₁ (modified chest lead) place the electrode discs as shown here: the ground electrode at the right shoulder, the negative electrode at the left shoulder, and the positive electrode at the sternal border.
2. Make sure the disc has enough gel to conduct the heart's electrical impulses.

for precordial V₁; the negative electrode in the clavicular hollow of the left shoulder; and the ground electrode in the clavicular hollow of the right shoulder (see photo 1).

Once you've located these sites, prepare the patient's skin for electrode attachment. First shave 4 inches around each site and clean with alcohol to remove skin oil. Allow to dry thoroughly. If the patient is sweating, apply a commercial antiperspirant spray or tincture of benzoin.

Nearly all electrode discs come prepackaged and pre-gelled. After opening the disc, check it carefully for adequate gel (see photo 2). If the gel has dried out, get a new disc. Apply all three discs on the designated sites and make sure the adhesive gives a tight seal. Be sure to apply them in the clavicular hollows; applying them over muscles risks interference from muscle tremors and patient movement.

Next, snap the small electrode cables (lead-

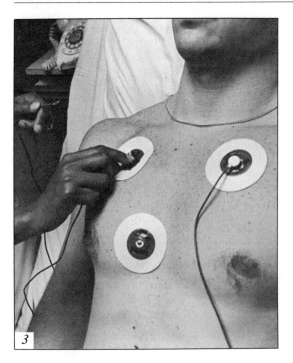

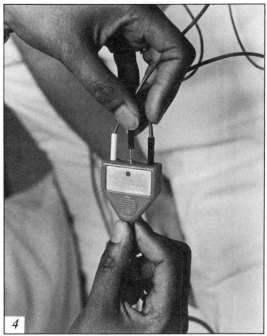

wire — photo 3) to the discs. Finally, insert the small electrode cables in the proper receptacles in the monitor cable (see photo 4). Be sure to insert the negative cable in the receptacle marked "—," "N," or "RA" (right arm); the positive cable in the receptacle marked "+," "P," or "LL" (left leg); and the ground cable into the receptacle marked "G" (ground) or "N" (neutral).

Although MCL₁ is the best lead for standard monitoring, you may want further information from other leads. Leave the ground and negative electrodes in place and simply move the positive electrode to another position. For example, to monitor a modified precordial V₆ lead, simply move the positive electrode to the left fifth intercostal space at the mid-axillary line.

If your patient is a likely candidate for arrhythmias such as bundle branch blocks or ectopic beats, you can attach several electrode discs at lead locations across his chest. Then, to

3. Snap the small electrode cables or leadwires to the electrode discs.
4. When connecting the lead wires to the monitor cable, be sure to insert the negative, positive, and ground lead wires in the proper receptacles.

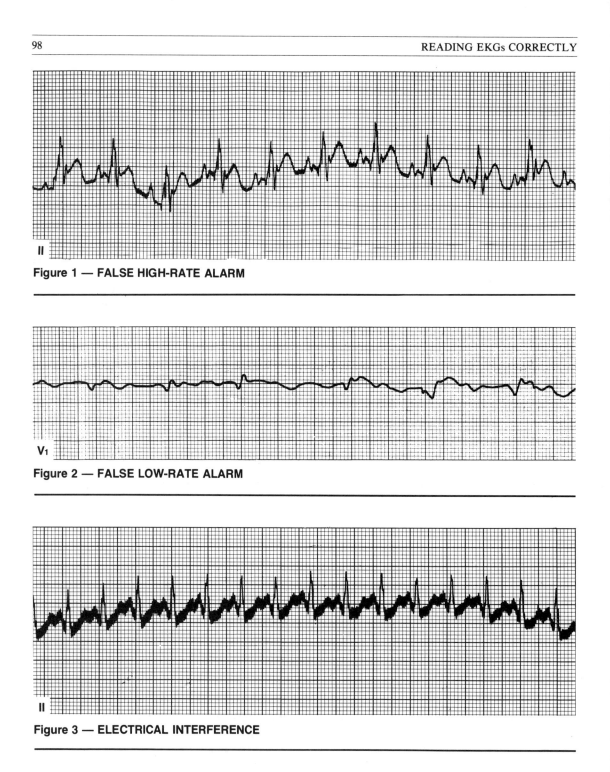

Figure 1 — FALSE HIGH-RATE ALARM

Figure 2 — FALSE LOW-RATE ALARM

Figure 3 — ELECTRICAL INTERFERENCE

quickly switch from one lead to another, just move the positive electrode cable from disc to disc.

Once you've started monitoring, periodically check the condition of the electrode discs. If the discs cause itching or irritation, change them to new sites near the previous sites. If they become loose, reapply them. If they still won't stick, replace them.

Tips on troubleshooting

Even minor disturbances in the monitoring system — electrical interference, loose electrodes, patient movement, and so forth — can create major interference with the EKG tracing. That is why you should learn to identify and quickly correct the most common monitor problems. Naturally your first step whenever you notice an artifact in a tracing should be to check the patient for medical causes. But if his condition appears stable, check for mechanical causes.

False high-rate alarm. As we've explained, the rate alarm averages the number of heart beats per minute by counting the QRS complexes. But if a tracing contains tall waves from sources other than the heart, the monitor will probably record them as QRS complexes and falsely sound the high-rate alarm.

One possible cause of a false high-rate alarm is skeletal muscle activity (muscle potential), which causes tall waves in a tracing (see Figure 1). To avoid this, apply electrodes away from large muscle masses, such as the pectoral muscles.

Another possible cause is T waves as tall as, or taller than, the QRS complexes. Once you've ruled out hyperkalemia as the cause for abnormally high T waves, check for other problems with the monitor. Try repositioning the electrodes to a different site. If the T waves are still too tall, turn the lead selector to a different lead — one where the QRS complexes have a higher amplitude than the T waves.

If the alarm persists, carefully check the system for: loose electrodes, damaged or broken wires or cables, improper connection of the cables. If these defects aren't causing the alarm, you may have set the alarm system too close to the patient's normal pulse rate. Check with the doctor.

False low-rate alarm. If the contact between skin and electrodes is insufficient to transmit electrical impulses, a false low rate will be recorded on the rate meter and sound the low-rate alarm. In some cases, the tracing may resemble idioventricular rhythm (Figure 2); or, it may resemble asystole. First, *check the patient*. If he doesn't seem to be in distress, check the electrodes. Chances are you'll find at least one of them making poor contact with the skin.

A second possible cause of a false low-rate alarm is patient movement. When a patient turns on his side, for instance, the axis of his heart shifts slightly, reducing the QRS amplitude. Since the rate meter can't detect the smaller QRS complexes, the low-rate alarm sounds.

If this happens, do not disturb the patient by asking him to change position; simply reset the gain knob to enlarge the QRS complexes.

If you're getting a baseline but no tracing, check the gain knob and the lead selector control to make sure they're positioned properly. If they are, also check the cable connections. If the connections are firm, finally check the cables for damage and have a service technician check the monitor for defects.

Electrical interference. Interference caused by electrical external voltage (60-cycle alternating current) appears on the oscilloscope and rhythm strip as a widened baseline (Figure 3). Not only does electrical interference distort the EKG and hide parts of the cardiac cycle; it also can indicate an electrical hazard to the patient and staff.

Since the main source of electrical interfer-

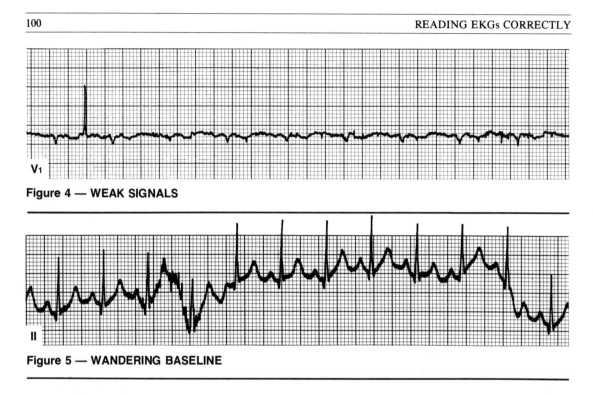

Figure 4 — WEAK SIGNALS

Figure 5 — WANDERING BASELINE

ence is improper grounding, ask the electrician to check the third prong in the power plug to make sure it's a true ground. Also move nearby electrical devices away from the monitor if at all possible. Sometimes you can eliminate 60-cycle interference simply by replacing the electrodes.

Weak signals. Indistinct or defective patterns on a monitor (see Figure 4) may result from improper setting of the gain dial, from poor electrode contact with the skin, from improper connection of the small electrode cables, or from malfunction of the monitor. Without question, though, the most common causes are improper setting of the gain dial and faulty contact between electrode and skin.

To correct weak signals, first try turning up the gain dial. If this doesn't improve the tracing, look for improper attachment of electrodes, too little or too much electrode jelly, and moist skin from sweating. If these are causing weak signals, reapply the electrodes.

Wandering baseline. If electrode connections are inadequate or if the electrodes move during patient movement or respiration, the monitor may register a wandering baseline (Figure 5).

When this occurs, first see if the patient's movement has disturbed the electrode connection. Also check to make sure tension on the cable isn't pulling the electrode from the patient's body. Be sure the cable is secured to the patient's gown. If that's not the problem, look to see if the patient's respiratory movements are loosening the electrodes from the skin. If so, move those electrodes to another part of the chest. If none of these checks reveals the cause of the wandering baseline, you can assume that it's being caused by external voltage variations; call the engineer.

Some final reminders

Cardiac monitors and electrocardiographs, through continuous surveillance, can give you priceless information. Not only can they help you assess arrhythmias that need definite therapy, even lifesaving measures; they also can help you gauge the effectiveness of therapy.

But monitors and electrocardiographs cannot replace you, the nurse. Only by deliberately and systematically checking clinical signs and symptoms and correlating them with your EKG findings can you truly assess a patient's condition. Remember that EKG interpretation is merely a tool of medicine. And like any tool, it's worthless unless you know how to use it correctly.

SKILLCHECK 10
The following tracings illustrate a few of the monitor problems discussed in this chapter. Try to diagnosis each problem, then determine the probable cause.

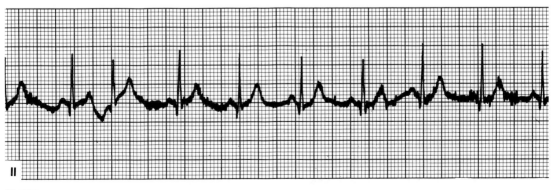

V₁

Problem _____

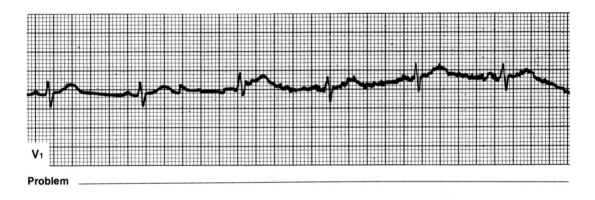

II

Problem _____

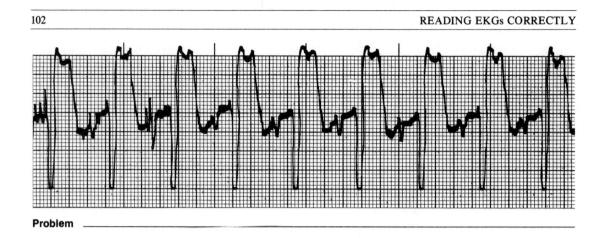

Problem

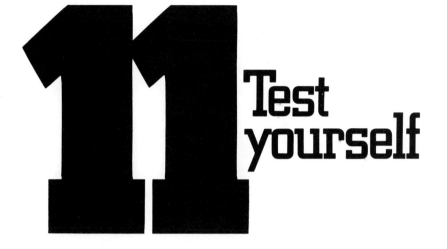

11 Test yourself

If you've faithfully read the preceding chapters, carefully studied the sample tracings, and diligently worked the skillchecks at the end of each chapter, you should have a working knowledge of EKG interpretation. Now, you must perfect your interpretation skills. And the only way to do that is to practice, practice, practice.

On the following pages you'll find numerous tracings that will give you an opportunity to do just that. As in real life, many have several answers. Be sure to study them carefully and record every finding.

As you go through these tracings, remember that they are self-tests — not a teacher's test. Our sole purpose in including them is to let you measure your progress and determine your strengths and weaknesses so *you* can decide where you need further study.

If one of your answers disagrees with the given answer, don't simply accept it as a mistake and go on to the next tracing. Instead, rework the tracing. Are your measurements accurate? Is the diagnosis consistent with those measurements? If your answer still disagrees with the given answer, reread the appropriate chapter and study the appropriate sample tracings. Are your measurements consistent with the criteria given for the sample tracings?

If, after scrutiny and research, your answer still seems correct and yet still disagrees with the given answer, you may have hit upon a tracing whose diagnosis is open to debate. Remember that EKG interpretation isn't an exact science. Even world-famous cardiologists have been known to disagree over the interpretation of some tracings, such as PACs and PNCs. The best you can do is to explore every possibility, to make sure your measurements are accurate, and to make the most logical, plausible interpretation.

After you've determined the correct diagnosis, we suggest you try to answer the key questions presented in chapter 2: Where did the arrhythmia originate? What is the heart doing?

What treatment might be needed to correct the arrhythmia, and what problems might that treatment create? What would happen to the patient if the arrhythmia were not treated? What special nursing considerations are implied by this arrhythmia? If you are unsure how to answer those questions for any specific arrhythmias, reread the appropriate chapters and study the criteria and treatment information listed under the sample strips. Only by answering all of these questions can you get the full value from the self tests.

One final word: This chapter is the end of the teaching portion of this book. But it should be only the beginning of your learning. Because you must constantly practice the skills you've learned here if you want to become truly proficient at EKG interpretation.

A striking example of the benefits of practice is the experience of a young nurse who attended our EKG lecture series several years ago. After each session, she begged for more information and for additional rhythm strips to analyze. She read several books on EKG interpretation outside class and pestered our EKG technician for old tracings. Even after our lecture series ended, she continued interpreting every tracing she could get her hands on.

A year later, she transferred to the coronary care unit at a larger teaching hospital. The chief cardiologist, after working with her for several weeks, commended her on her ability to analyze tracings, which compared favorably with that of most interns' and residents'. Even though she hadn't had any formal management training, he recommended her for promotion to head nurse in CCU.

Today, she has been head nurse for almost four years. Her hard work, and lots of practice, paid off.

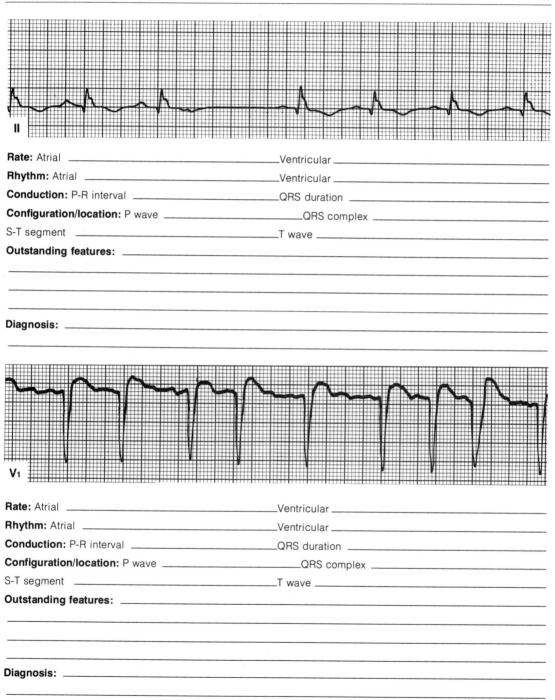

II

Rate: Atrial _____ Ventricular _____

Rhythm: Atrial _____ Ventricular _____

Conduction: P-R interval _____ QRS duration _____

Configuration/location: P wave _____ QRS complex _____

S-T segment _____ T wave _____

Outstanding features: _____

_____

_____

_____

Diagnosis: _____

_____

V₁

Rate: Atrial _____ Ventricular _____

Rhythm: Atrial _____ Ventricular _____

Conduction: P-R interval _____ QRS duration _____

Configuration/location: P wave _____ QRS complex _____

S-T segment _____ T wave _____

Outstanding features: _____

_____

_____

Diagnosis: _____

_____

(See next page for answers.)

Rate: Atrial — 75   Ventricular — 75

Rhythm: Atrial — *Regular*   Ventricular — *Regular (one dropped QRS)*

Conduction: P-R — *0.24 sec.*   QRS duration — *0.14 sec.*

Configuration/location: P wave — *Configuration varies; precedes QRS.*   QRS complex — *Wide, prolonged.*   S-T segment — *Normal.*   T wave — *Inverted*

Outstanding features: *One dropped QRS. Conduction delay through AV node and bundle branches. Varying configuration of P waves. Inverted T waves.*

Diagnosis: *Normal sinus rhythm; nonconducted PAC; first degree heart block*

Rate: Atrial — *Approximately 500*   Ventricular — *Approximately 100*

Rhythm: Atrial — *Chaotic*   Ventricular — *Irregular*

Conduction: P-R — *Not measurable*   QRS duration — *0.14 sec.*

Configuration/location: P wave — *Merged with T waves.*   QRS complex — *Normal; wide.*   S-T segment — *Elevated.*   T wave — *Merged with P waves.*

Outstanding features: *Rapid atrial rate. Normal ventricular rate. Irregular atrial and ventricular rhythms. Wide QRS.*

Diagnosis: *Atrial fibrillation; ventricular conduction delay*

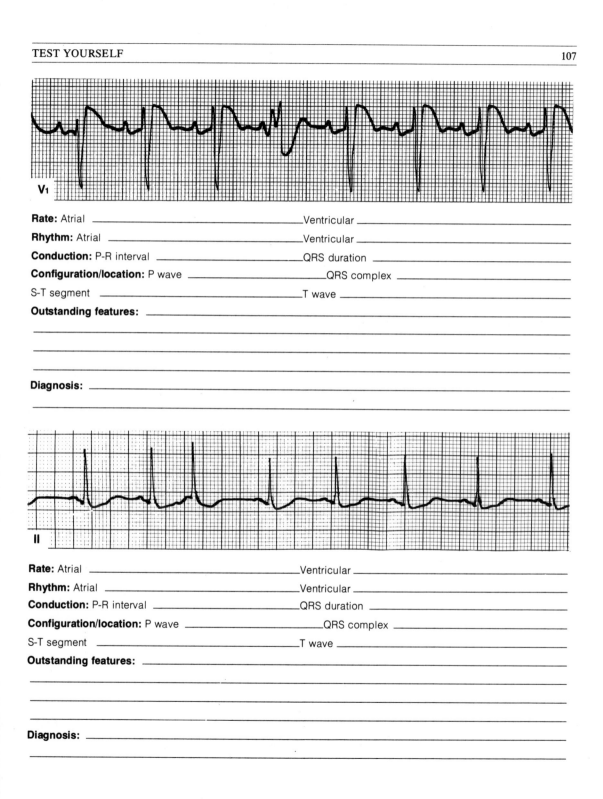

V₁

Rate: Atrial _____ Ventricular _____

Rhythm: Atrial _____ Ventricular _____

Conduction: P-R interval _____ QRS duration _____

Configuration/location: P wave _____ QRS complex _____

S-T segment _____ T wave _____

Outstanding features: _____

_____

_____

_____

Diagnosis: _____

_____

II

Rate: Atrial _____ Ventricular _____

Rhythm: Atrial _____ Ventricular _____

Conduction: P-R interval _____ QRS duration _____

Configuration/location: P wave _____ QRS complex _____

S-T segment _____ T wave _____

Outstanding features: _____

_____

_____

_____

Diagnosis: _____

_____

Rate: Atrial — *79*   Ventricular — *79*

Rhythm: Atrial — *Regular*   Ventricular — *Regular*

Conduction: P-R — *0.20 sec.*   QRS duration — *0.12 sec.*

Configuration/location: P wave — *Normal; precedes QRS.*   QRS complex — *Slightly widened.* S-T segment —
Elevated.   T wave — *Rounded.*

Outstanding features: *Normal rates. Normal atrial and ventricular rhythms. Prolonged QRS duration.*

Diagnosis: *Normal sinus rhythm; PVC*

Rate: Atrial — *75*   Ventricular — *75*

Rhythm: Atrial — *Slightly irregular*   Ventricular — *Slightly irregular*

Conduction: P-R — *0.16 sec.*   QRS duration — *0.10 sec.*

Configuration/location: P wave — *Changes configuration; precedes QRS.*   QRS complex — *Normal.*   S-T segment
— *Slightly depressed.*   T wave — *Rounded.*

Outstanding features: *Slightly irregular atrial and ventricular rhythms. P-R intervals vary slightly. P wave changes
configuration.*

Diagnosis: *Wandering pacemaker with junctional premature beats*

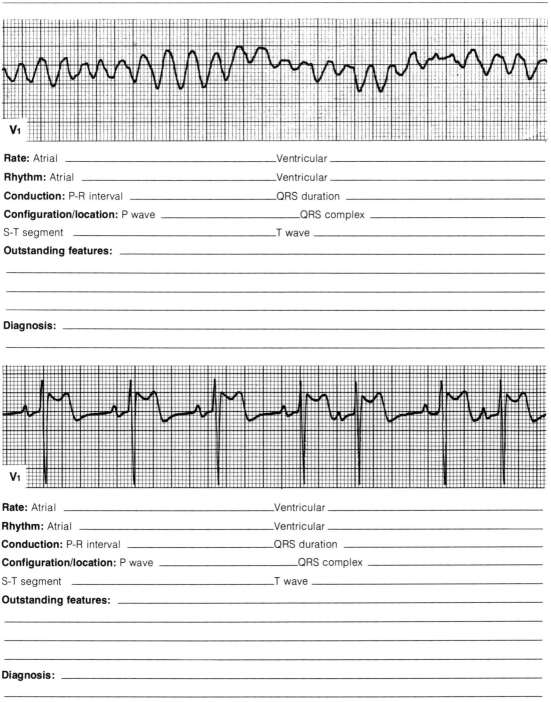

V₁

Rate: Atrial _____Ventricular _____

Rhythm: Atrial _____Ventricular _____

Conduction: P-R interval _____QRS duration _____

Configuration/location: P wave _____QRS complex _____

S-T segment _____T wave _____

Outstanding features: _____

_____

_____

_____

Diagnosis: _____

_____

V₁

Rate: Atrial _____Ventricular _____

Rhythm: Atrial _____Ventricular _____

Conduction: P-R interval _____QRS duration _____

Configuration/location: P wave _____QRS complex _____

S-T segment _____T wave _____

Outstanding features: _____

_____

_____

_____

Diagnosis: _____

_____

Rate: Atrial — *Not measurable*   Ventricular — *Not measurable*

Rhythm: Atrial — *Not measurable*   Ventricular — *Not measurable*

Conduction: P-R — *Not measurable*   QRS duration — *Not measurable*

Configuration/location: P wave — *Absent.*   QRS complex — *Absent.*   S-T segment — *Absent.*   T wave — *Absent.*

Outstanding features: *Chaotic baseline.*

Diagnosis: *Coarse ventricular fibrillation*

Rate: Atrial — *65*   Ventricular — *65*

Rhythm: Atrial — *Regular*   Ventricular — *Regular with some short cycles*

Conduction: P-R — *0.20 sec.*   QRS duration — *0.10 sec.*

Configuration/location: P wave — *Normal; precedes QRS.*   QRS complex — *Normal.*   S-T segment — *Elevated.*   T wave — *Peaked.*

Outstanding features: *Normal atrial and ventricular rates. Irregular ventricular rhythm (short cycles).*

Diagnosis: *Normal sinus rhythm with premature atrial contraction*

II

Rate: Atrial _____ Ventricular _____

Rhythm: Atrial _____ Ventricular _____

Conduction: P-R interval _____ QRS duration _____

Configuration/location: P wave _____ QRS complex _____

S-T segment _____ T wave _____

Outstanding features: _____

_____

_____

Diagnosis: _____

_____

V1

Rate: Atrial _____ Ventricular _____

Rhythm: Atrial _____ Ventricular _____

Conduction: P-R interval _____ QRS duration _____

Configuration/location: P wave _____ QRS complex _____

S-T segment _____ T wave _____

Outstanding features: _____

_____

_____

Diagnosis: _____

_____

Rate: Atrial — *46*   Ventricular — *46*

Rhythm: Atrial — *Regular*   Ventricular — *Regular*

Conduction: P-R — *0.16 sec.*   QRS duration — *0.08 sec.*

Configuration/location: P wave — *Normal; precedes QRS.*   QRS complex — *Normal; follows P wave.*   S-T segment — *Normal.*   T wave — *Slightly flat*

Outstanding features: *Slow atrial and ventricular rates.*

Diagnosis: *Sinus bradycardia*

Rate: Atrial — *Not measurable*   Ventricular — *Approximately 100*

Rhythm: Atrial — *Irregular*   Ventricular— *Irregular*

Conduction: P-R — *0.12 sec.*   QRS duration — *0.10 sec.*

Configuration/location: P wave — *Normal when present; every other one precedes QRS.*   QRS complex — *Normal.*   S-T segment — *Slightly elevated.*   T wave — *Every other one wide and round.*

Outstanding features: *Every other QRS complex not preceded by a P wave. In these cycles, apparent merging of T waves with a premature P wave.*

Diagnosis: *Atrial bigeminy*

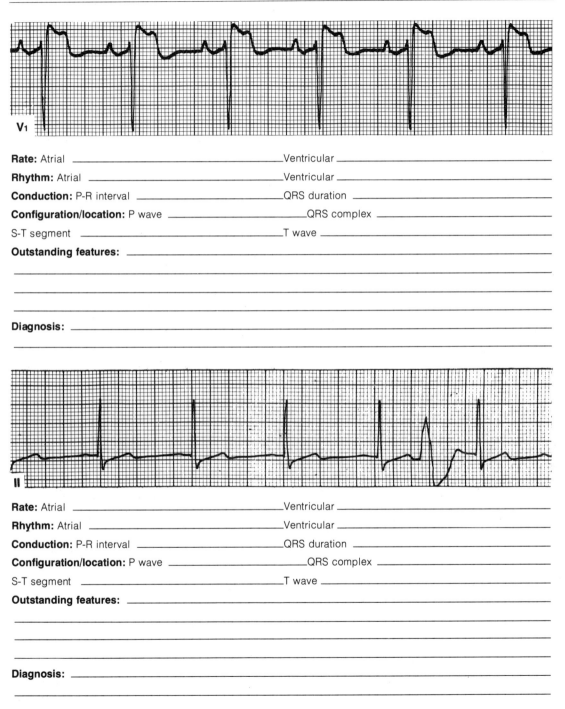

V₁

Rate: Atrial _____ Ventricular _____

Rhythm: Atrial _____ Ventricular _____

Conduction: P-R interval _____ QRS duration _____

Configuration/location: P wave _____ QRS complex _____

S-T segment _____ T wave _____

Outstanding features: _____

_____

_____

Diagnosis: _____

_____

II

Rate: Atrial _____ Ventricular _____

Rhythm: Atrial _____ Ventricular _____

Conduction: P-R interval _____ QRS duration _____

Configuration/location: P wave _____ QRS complex _____

S-T segment _____ T wave _____

Outstanding features: _____

_____

_____

Diagnosis: _____

_____

Rate: Atrial — *Approximately 60*   Ventricular — *Approximately 60*

Rhythm: Atrial — *Slightly irregular*   Ventricular — *Slightly irregular*

Conduction: P-R — *0.24 sec.*   QRS duration — *0.10 sec.*

Configuration/location: P wave — *Normal; precedes QRS.*   QRS complex — *Normal; follows P.*   S-T segment — *Elevated.*   T wave — *Rounded.*

Outstanding features: *Slow atrial and ventricular rate. Slightly irregular atrial and ventricular rhythms. Prolonged P-R interval (A-V conduction delay).*

Diagnosis: *Sinus bradycardia; sinus arrhythmia; first degree heart block*

Rate: Atrial — *60*   Ventricular — *60*

Rhythm: Atrial — *Regular*   Ventricular — *Slightly irregular*

Conduction: P-R — *0.20 sec.*   QRS duration — *0.10 sec.*

Configuration/location: P wave — *Flat; precedes QRS.*   QRS complex — *Normal.*   S-T segment — *Depressed.*   T wave — *Rounding.*

Outstanding features: *Slow atrial and ventricular rates. Regular atrial rhythm; irregular ventricular rhythm. One wide, bizarre QRS.*

Diagnosis: *Sinus bradycardia, PVC interpolated*

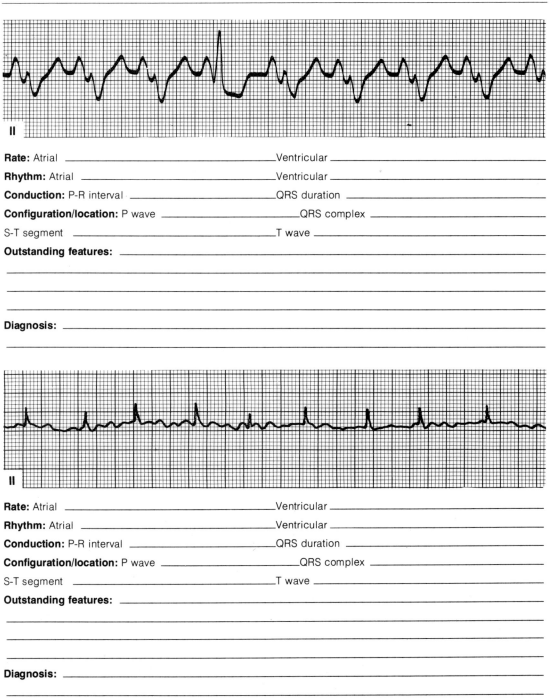

Rate: Atrial _____ Ventricular _____

Rhythm: Atrial _____ Ventricular _____

Conduction: P-R interval _____ QRS duration _____

Configuration/location: P wave _____ QRS complex _____

S-T segment _____ T wave _____

Outstanding features: _____

_____

_____

_____

Diagnosis: _____

_____

Rate: Atrial _____ Ventricular _____

Rhythm: Atrial _____ Ventricular _____

Conduction: P-R interval _____ QRS duration _____

Configuration/location: P wave _____ QRS complex _____

S-T segment _____ T wave _____

Outstanding features: _____

_____

_____

_____

Diagnosis: _____

_____

Rate: Atrial — *83*   Ventricular — *83*

Rhythm: Atrial — *Regular*   Ventricular — *Regular*

Conduction: P-R — *0.16 sec.*   QRS duration — *0.22 sec.*

Configuration/location: P wave — *Peaked; precedes most QRS.*   QRS complex — *Wide.*   S-T segment — *Elevated.*   T wave — *Normal.*

Outstanding features: *Normal atrial and ventricular rates. Regular atrial and ventricular rhythms. Wide QRS complex; one distorted.*

Diagnosis: *Normal sinus rhythm with PVC and right bundle branch block*

Rate: Atrial — *Approximately 500*   Ventricular — *Approximately 88*

Rhythm: Atrial — *Irregular*   Ventricular — *Irregular*

Conduction: P-R — *Not measurable*   QRS duration — *0.08 sec.*

Configuration/location: P wave — *Merged with T wave.*   QRS complex — *Normal.*   S-T segment — *Not measurable.*   T wave — *Merged with P wave.*

Outstanding features: *Rapid atrial rate. Irregular ventricular rhythm. No P or T waves. No measurable P-R interval.*

Diagnosis: *Atrial fibrillation*

V₁

Rate: Atrial _____ Ventricular _____

Rhythm: Atrial _____ Ventricular _____

Conduction: P-R interval _____ QRS duration _____

Configuration/location: P wave _____ QRS complex _____

S-T segment _____ T wave _____

Outstanding features: _____

_____

_____

Diagnosis: _____

II

Rate: Atrial _____ Ventricular _____

Rhythm: Atrial _____ Ventricular _____

Conduction: P-R interval _____ QRS duration _____

Configuration/location: P wave _____ QRS complex _____

S-T segment _____ T wave _____

Outstanding features: _____

_____

_____

Diagnosis: _____

Rate: Atrial — *Not measurable*   Ventricular — *250*

Rhythm: Atrial — *Not measurable*   Ventricular — *Regular*

Conduction: P-R — *Not measurable*   QRS — *0.24 sec.*

Configuration/location: P wave — *Absent.*   QRS complex — *Wide and bizarre.*   S-T segment — *None.*   T wave — *Absent.*

Outstanding features: *Chaotic baseline. No discernible complexes.*

Diagnosis: *Ventricular tachycardia*

Rate: Atrial — *Not measurable*   Ventricular — *72*

Rhythm: Atrial — *Not measurable*   Ventricular — *Regular*

Conduction: P-R — *Not measurable*   QRS duration — *0.08 sec.*

Configuration/location: P wave — *Absent.*   QRS complex — *Normal.*   S-T segment — *Depressed.*   T wave — *Rounded*

Outstanding features: *Absent P waves. Regular ventricular rhythm.*

Diagnosis: *Junctional tachycardia*

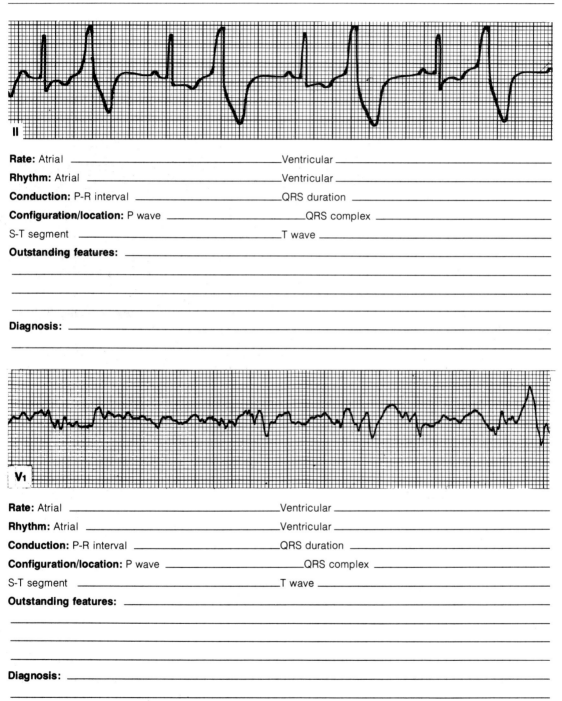

II

Rate: Atrial _____ Ventricular _____

Rhythm: Atrial _____ Ventricular _____

Conduction: P-R interval _____ QRS duration _____

Configuration/location: P wave _____ QRS complex _____

S-T segment _____ T wave _____

Outstanding features: _____

_____

_____

_____

Diagnosis: _____

_____

V₁

Rate: Atrial _____ Ventricular _____

Rhythm: Atrial _____ Ventricular _____

Conduction: P-R interval _____ QRS duration _____

Configuration/location: P wave _____ QRS complex _____

S-T segment _____ T wave _____

Outstanding features: _____

_____

_____

_____

Diagnosis: _____

_____

Rate: Atrial — *Not measurable*   Ventricular — *43*

Rhythm: Atrial — *Not measurable*   Ventricular — *Irregular*

Conduction: P-R — *0.18 sec.*   QRS duration — *0.12 sec.*

Configuration/location: P wave — *Rounded; precedes some QRS.*   QRS complex — *Distorted.*   S-T segment —

Depressed.   T wave — *Inverted.*

Outstanding features: *Slow ventricular rate. Unable to determine atrial rate. Every other QRS distorted;*

wide and bizarre.

Diagnosis: *Ventricular bigeminy*

Rate: Atrial — *Not measurable*   Ventricular — *Not measurable*

Rhythm: Atrial — *Not measurable*   Ventricular — *Not measurable*

Conduction: P-R — *Not measurable*   QRS duration — *Not measurable*

Configuration/location: P wave — *Absent.*   QRS complex — *Absent.*   S-T segment — *Absent.*   T wave — *Absent.*

Outstanding features: *Undulating, chaotic baseline. No distinguishing features.*

Diagnosis: *Ventricular fibrillation*

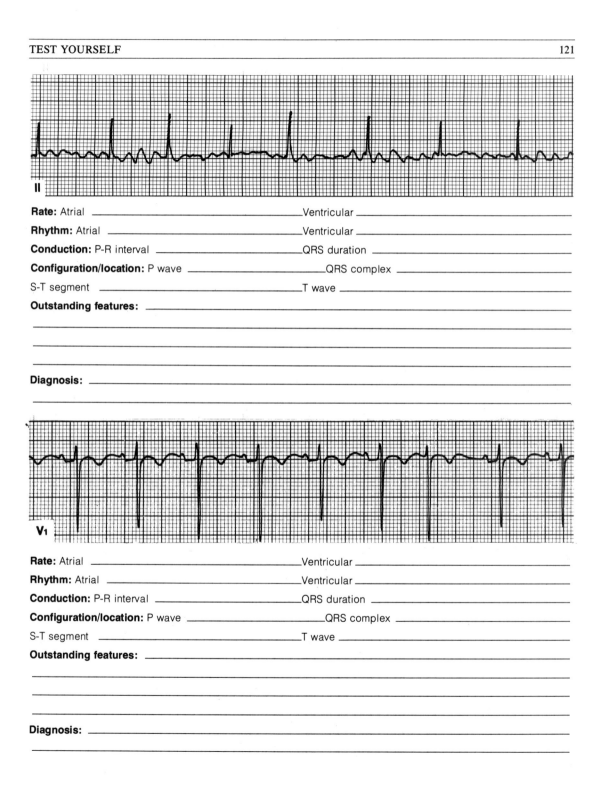

II

Rate: Atrial _____ Ventricular _____

Rhythm: Atrial _____ Ventricular _____

Conduction: P-R interval _____ QRS duration _____

Configuration/location: P wave _____ QRS complex _____

S-T segment _____ T wave _____

Outstanding features: _____
_____
_____
_____

Diagnosis: _____
_____

V₁

Rate: Atrial _____ Ventricular _____

Rhythm: Atrial _____ Ventricular _____

Conduction: P-R interval _____ QRS duration _____

Configuration/location: P wave _____ QRS complex _____

S-T segment _____ T wave _____

Outstanding features: _____
_____
_____
_____

Diagnosis: _____
_____

Rate: Atrial — *375*   Ventricular — *Approximately 75*

Rhythm: Atrial — *Irregular*   Ventricular — *Irregular*

Conduction: P-R — *Not measurable*   QRS duration — *0.08 sec.*

Configuration/location: P wave — *Lost in T wave.*   QRS complex — *Normal.*   S-T segment — *Not measurable.*   T wave — *Merged with P wave.*

Outstanding features: *Rapid atrial rate. Ventricular rate slower than atrial rate. No measurable P-R interval. Irregular atrial and ventricular rhythms. P waves and T waves merged to form uneven baseline.*

Diagnosis: *Atrial flutter – fibrillation ("flutteration")*

Rate: Atrial — *88*   Ventricular — *88*

Rhythm: Atrial — *Regular*   Ventricular — *Regular with one short cycle*

Conduction: P-R — *0.16 sec.*   QRS duration — *0.08 sec.*

Configuration/location: P wave — *Normal; precedes QRS.*   QRS complex — *Normal; follows P wave.*   S-T segment — *Slightly elevated.*   T wave — *Inverted.*

Outstanding features: *Normal atrial and ventricular rates. Regular atrial rhythm. Regular ventricular rhythm with one short cycle.*

Diagnosis: *Normal sinus rhythm with premature atrial contraction*

V₁

Rate: Atrial _____ Ventricular _____

Rhythm: Atrial _____ Ventricular _____

Conduction: P-R interval _____ QRS duration _____

Configuration/location: P wave _____ QRS complex _____

S-T segment _____ T wave _____

Outstanding features: _____

_____

_____

Diagnosis: _____

_____

V₁

Rate: Atrial _____ Ventricular _____

Rhythm: Atrial _____ Ventricular _____

Conduction: P-R interval _____ QRS duration _____

Configuration/location: P wave _____ QRS complex _____

S-T segment _____ T wave _____

Outstanding features: _____

_____

_____

Diagnosis: _____

_____

Rate: Atrial — *83*   Ventricular — *83*

Rhythm: Atrial — *Irregular*   Ventricular — *Irregular*

Conduction: P-R — *0.20 sec.*   QRS duration — *0.10 sec.*

Configuration/location: P wave — *Normal; precedes QRS.*   QRS complex — *Normal; follows P.*   S-T segment — *Elevated.*   T wave — *Rounded.*

Outstanding features: *Slightly irregular atrial and ventricular rhythms. Long pause with dropped QRS complex that was not preceded by a P wave. One short R-R interval with P-R intervals less than patient's normal P-R.*

Diagnosis: *Normal sinus rhythm; premature atrial contraction; sinus arrest*

Rate: Atrial — *Not measurable*   Ventricular — *Not measurable*

Rhythm: Atrial — *Not measurable*   Ventricular — *Not measurable*

Conduction: P-R — *Not measurable*   QRS duration — *Not measurable*

Configuration/location: P wave — *Not visible.*   QRS complex — *Not measurable.*   S-T segment — *Not measurable.*   T wave — *Not measurable.*

Outstanding features: *Chaotic rhythm with no discernible characteristics.*

Diagnosis: *Ventricular fibrillation*

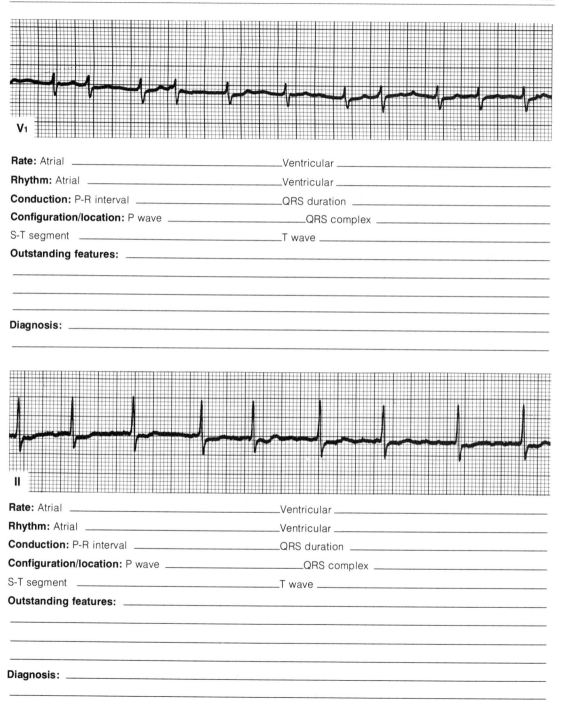

V₁

Rate: Atrial _____ Ventricular _____

Rhythm: Atrial _____ Ventricular _____

Conduction: P-R interval _____ QRS duration _____

Configuration/location: P wave _____ QRS complex _____

S-T segment _____ T wave _____

Outstanding features: _____

_____

_____

_____

Diagnosis: _____

_____

II

Rate: Atrial _____ Ventricular _____

Rhythm: Atrial _____ Ventricular _____

Conduction: P-R interval _____ QRS duration _____

Configuration/location: P wave _____ QRS complex _____

S-T segment _____ T wave _____

Outstanding features: _____

_____

_____

_____

Diagnosis: _____

_____

Rate: Atrial — *Approximately 500*   Ventricular — *Approximately 115*

Rhythm: Atrial — *Irregular*   Ventricular — *Irregular*

Conduction: P-R — *Not measurable*   QRS duration — *0.10 sec.*

Configuration/location: P wave — *Merged with T waves.*   QRS complex — *Widened.*   S-T segment — *Normal.*   T wave — *Merged with P waves.*

Outstanding features: *Rapid atrial rate. Slightly rapid ventricular rate. Irregular atrial and ventricular rhythms.*

Diagnosis: *Atrial fibrillation*

Rate: Atrial — *Approximately 500*   Ventricular — *Approximately 88*

Rhythm: Atrial — *Irregular*   Ventricular — *Irregular*

Conduction: P-R — *Not measurable*   QRS duration — *0.10 sec.*

Configuration/location: P wave — *Merged with T wave.*   QRS complex — *Normal.*   S-T segment — *Slightly depressed.*   T wave — *Merged with P wave.*

Outstanding features: *Rapid atrial rate. Irregular atrial and ventricular rhythms. Merged P and T waves.*

Diagnosis: *Atrial fibrillation*

III

Rate: Atrial _____ Ventricular _____

Rhythm: Atrial _____ Ventricular _____

Conduction: P-R interval _____ QRS duration _____

Configuration/location: P wave _____ QRS complex _____

S-T segment _____ T wave _____

Outstanding features: _____

_____

_____

_____

Diagnosis: _____

_____

II

Rate: Atrial _____ Ventricular _____

Rhythm: Atrial _____ Ventricular _____

Conduction: P-R interval _____ QRS duration _____

Configuration/location: P wave _____ QRS complex _____

S-T segment _____ T wave _____

Outstanding features: _____

_____

_____

_____

Diagnosis: _____

_____

Rate: Atrial — *79*   Ventricular — *79*

Rhythm: Atrial — *Regular*   Ventricular — *Regular*

Conduction: P-R — *0.24 sec.*   QRS duration — *0.16 sec.*

Configuration/location: P wave — *Normal; precedes QRS.*   QRS complex — *Wide; follows P waves.*   S-T segment — *Normal.*   T wave — *Inverted.*

Outstanding features: *Normal atrial and ventricular rates. Regular atrial and ventricular rhythms. Prolonged P-R interval and QRS duration.*

Diagnosis: *Normal sinus rhythm; first degree block; PVC; right bundle branch block*

Rate: Atrial — *107*   Ventricular — *107*

Rhythm: Atrial — *Not measurable*   Ventricular — *Regular*

Conduction: P-R — *Not measurable*   QRS duration — *0.18 sec.*

Configuration/location: P wave — *Absent.*   QRS complex — *Normal.*   S-T segment — *Slightly depressed.*
T wave — *Inverted*

Outstanding features: *Absent P waves. Regular ventricular rhythm.*

Diagnosis: *Junctional tachycardia*

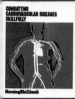

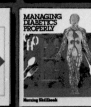
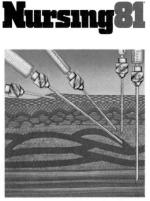

Choose one of these important books as your introductory volume when you join the NURSING SKILLBOOK series...the most comprehensive reference series ever published for nurses.

- Using Crisis Intervention Wisely • Coping With Neurologic Problems Proficiently
- Managing Diabetics Properly • Helping Cancer Patients Effectively
- Documenting Patient Care Responsibly • Monitoring Fluid and Electrolytes Precisely • Giving Cardiovascular Drugs Safely • Assessing Vital Functions Accurately • Nursing Critically Ill Patients Confidently • Giving Emergency Care Competently • Reading EKGs Correctly • Combatting Cardiovascular Diseases Skillfully • Dealing with Death and Dying

NO POSTAGE
NECESSARY
IF MAILED
IN THE
UNITED STATES

BUSINESS REPLY CARD
FIRST CLASS PERMIT NO. 1903 HICKSVILLE, N.Y.

POSTAGE WILL BE PAID BY ADDRESSEE

The
Skillbook
Company

6 Commercial Street
Hicksville, N.Y. 11801

NO POSTAGE
NECESSARY
IF MAILED
IN THE
UNITED STATES

BUSINESS REPLY CARD
FIRST CLASS PERMIT NO. 182 MANASQUAN, N.J.

POSTAGE WILL BE PAID BY ADDRESSEE

Nursing 81®

One Health Road
P.O. Box 1008
Manasquan, N.J. 08736

V₁

Rate: Atrial _____ Ventricular _____

Rhythm: Atrial _____ Ventricular _____

Conduction: P-R interval _____ QRS duration _____

Configuration/location: P wave _____ QRS complex _____

S-T segment _____ T wave _____

Outstanding features: _____

_____

_____

_____

Diagnosis: _____

_____

I

Rate: Atrial _____ Ventricular _____

Rhythm: Atrial _____ Ventricular _____

Conduction: P-R interval _____ QRS duration _____

Configuration/location: P wave _____ QRS complex _____

S-T segment _____ T wave _____

Outstanding features: _____

_____

_____

_____

Diagnosis: _____

_____

Rate: Atrial — *94*   Ventricular — *94*

Rhythm: Atrial — *Fairly regular*   Ventricular — *Irregular*

Conduction: P-R — *0.20 sec.*   QRS duration — *0.08 sec.*

Configuration/location: P wave — *Low; rounded; precedes most QRS.*   QRS complex — *Normal; 2 wide and distorted.*   S-T segment — *Elevated.*   T wave — *Rounded.*

Outstanding features: *Normal atrial and ventricular rates. Irregular ventricular rhythm. Two distorted and wide QRS complexes.*

Diagnosis: *Normal sinus rhythm with PVCs*

Rate: Atrial — *88*   Ventricular — *88*

Rhythm: Atrial — *Regular*   Ventricular — *Regular*

Conduction: P-R — *0.18 sec.*   QRS duration — *0.14 sec.*

Configuration/location: P wave — *Low; precedes QRS.*   QRS complex — *Wide; follows P wave.*   S-T segment — *Depressed.*   T wave — *Flat.*

Outstanding features: *Prolonged QRS duration.*

Diagnosis: *Normal sinus rhythm; left bundle branch block; anterior wall ischemia*

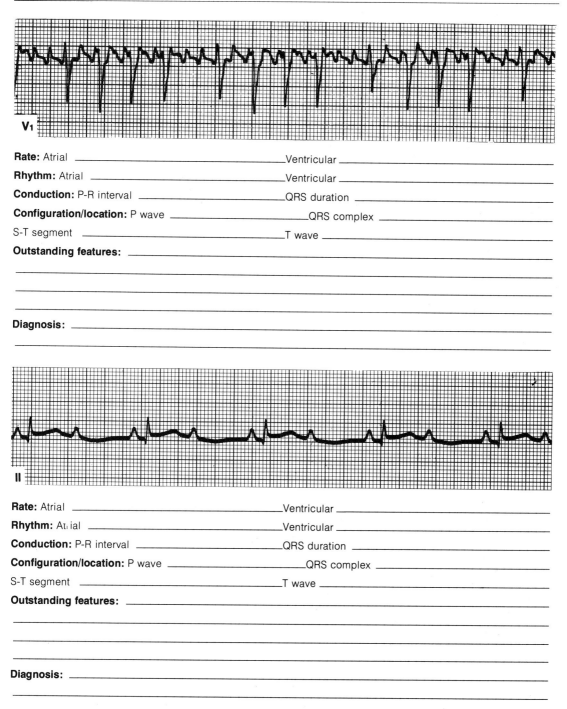

Rate: Atrial _____ Ventricular _____

Rhythm: Atrial _____ Ventricular _____

Conduction: P-R interval _____ QRS duration _____

Configuration/location: P wave _____ QRS complex _____

S-T segment _____ T wave _____

Outstanding features: _____

_____

_____

Diagnosis: _____

Rate: Atrial _____ Ventricular _____

Rhythm: Atrial _____ Ventricular _____

Conduction: P-R interval _____ QRS duration _____

Configuration/location: P wave _____ QRS complex _____

S-T segment _____ T wave _____

Outstanding features: _____

_____

_____

Diagnosis: _____

Rate: Atrial — *375*   Ventricular — *136*

Rhythm: Atrial — *Irregular*   Ventricular — *Irregular*

Conduction: P-R — *Not measurable*   QRS duration — *0.08 sec.*

Configuration/location: P wave — *Merged with T wave.*   QRS complex — *Normal.*   S-T segment — *Elevated.*   T wave — *Merged with P wave.*

Outstanding features: *Rapid atrial and ventricular rates. Irregular ventricular rhythm.*

Diagnosis: *Atrial flutter 2:1 and 4:1*

Rate: Atrial — *94*   Ventricular — *47*

Rhythm: Atrial — *Regular*   Ventricular — *Regular*

Conduction: P-R — *0.20 sec.*   QRS duration — *0.10 sec.*

Configuration/location: P wave — *Normal; precedes QRS.*   QRS complex — *Normal; some absent.*   S-T segment — *Elevated.*   T wave — *Rounded.*

Outstanding features: *Atrial rate twice the ventricular rate. Two P waves for every QRS complex. Consistent P-R interval.*

Diagnosis: *Second degree block 2:1*

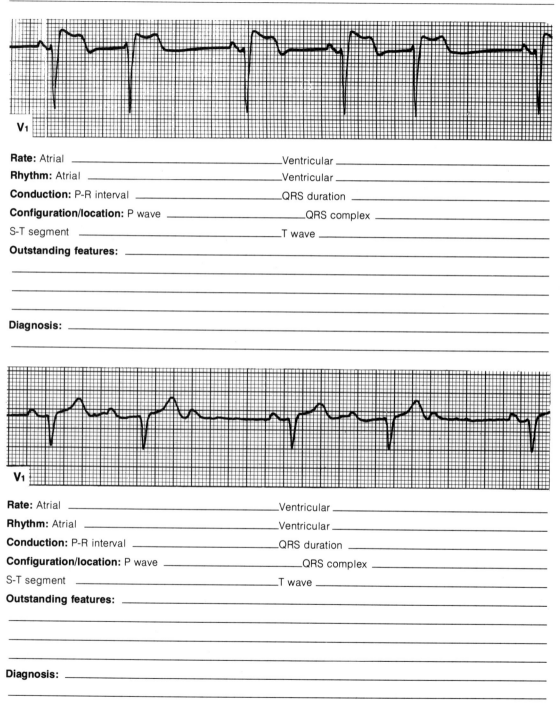

V1

Rate: Atrial _____ Ventricular _____

Rhythm: Atrial _____ Ventricular _____

Conduction: P-R interval _____ QRS duration _____

Configuration/location: P wave _____ QRS complex _____

S-T segment _____ T wave _____

Outstanding features: _____

_____

_____

_____

Diagnosis: _____

_____

V1

Rate: Atrial _____ Ventricular _____

Rhythm: Atrial _____ Ventricular _____

Conduction: P-R interval _____ QRS duration _____

Configuration/location: P wave _____ QRS complex _____

S-T segment _____ T wave _____

Outstanding features: _____

_____

_____

_____

Diagnosis: _____

_____

Rate: Atrial — *58*   Ventricular — *Approximately 58*

Rhythm: Atrial — *Irregular*   Ventricular — *Irregular*

Conduction: P-R — *0.16 sec.*   QRS duration — *0.12 sec.*

Configuration/location: P wave — *Normal; absent in shorter cycles.*   QRS complex — *Normal.*   S-T segment — *Elevated.*   T wave — *Normal*

Outstanding features: *Irregular ventricular rhythm caused by short cycles. P waves absent in short cycles.*

Diagnosis: *Normal sinus rhythm with premature junctional beats.*

Rate: Atrial — *72*   Ventricular — *39 to 63 (depends on block)*

Rhythm: Atrial — *Slightly irregular*   Ventricular — *Irregular*

Conduction: P-R — *Varies*   QRS duration — *0.12 sec.*

Configuration/location: P wave — *Rounded; precedes QRS.*   QRS complex — *Broad; some absent.*   S-T segment — *Elevated.*   T wave — *Rounded.*

Outstanding features: *Three P waves for every two QRS complexes. P-R varies. Ventricular rate and rhythm vary with degree of block.*

Diagnosis: *Second degree block – (Wenckebach 3:2 conduction)*

II

Rate: Atrial _____ Ventricular _____

Rhythm: Atrial _____ Ventricular _____

Conduction: P-R interval _____ QRS duration _____

Configuration/location: P wave _____ QRS complex _____

S-T segment _____ T wave _____

Outstanding features: _____

_____

_____

_____

Diagnosis: _____

_____

V₁

Rate: Atrial _____ Ventricular _____

Rhythm: Atrial _____ Ventricular _____

Conduction: P-R interval _____ QRS duration _____

Configuration/location: P wave _____ QRS complex _____

S-T segment _____ T wave _____

Outstanding features: _____

_____

_____

_____

Diagnosis: _____

_____

Rate: Atrial — *83*   Ventricular — *83*

Rhythm: Atrial — *Regular*   Ventricular — *Fairly regular*

Conduction: P-R — *0.18 sec.*   QRS duration — *0.12 sec.*

Configuration/location: P wave — *Some flat; some varying shapes; some absent; usually precede QRS.*   QRS complex — *Slightly wide, changes direction in some beats.*   S-T segment — *Depressed and elevated.*   T wave — *Rounded and peaked.*

Outstanding features: *Normal heart rates. Regular atrial rhythm. Slightly irregular ventricular rhythm. Prolonged QRS duration.*

Diagnosis: *Normal sinus rhythm; short run of ventricular tachycardia*

Rate: Atrial — *Approximately 500*   Ventricular — *Approximately 100*

Rhythm: Atrial — *Chaotic; irregular*   Ventricular — *Irregular*

Conduction: P-R — *Not measurable.*   QRS duration — *0.10 sec.*

Configuration/location: P wave — *Merged with T waves.*   QRS complex — *Normal.*   S-T segment — *Elevated.*   T wave — *Merged with P waves.*

Outstanding features: *Different atrial and ventricular rates. Irregular atrial rhythm (chaotic baseline). Irregular ventricular rhythm. Merged P waves and T waves to form "f" waves.*

Diagnosis: *Atrial fibrillation*

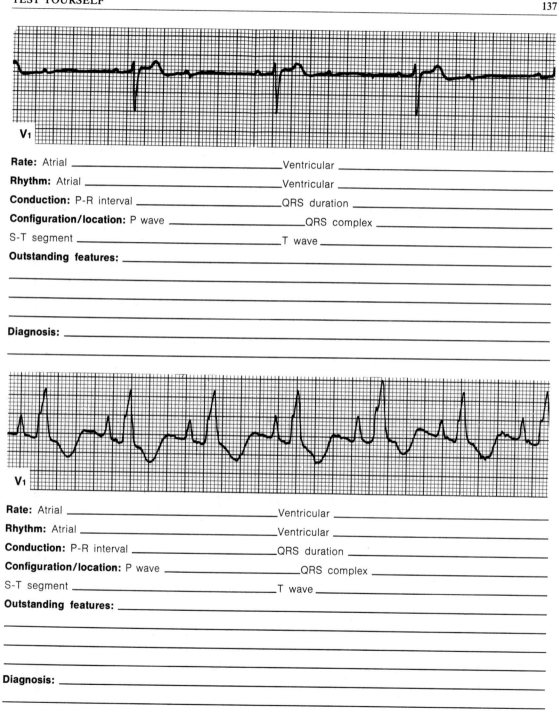

V₁

Rate: Atrial _____ Ventricular _____

Rhythm: Atrial _____ Ventricular _____

Conduction: P-R interval _____ QRS duration _____

Configuration/location: P wave _____ QRS complex _____

S-T segment _____ T wave _____

Outstanding features: _____
_____
_____
_____

Diagnosis: _____
_____

V₁

Rate: Atrial _____ Ventricular _____

Rhythm: Atrial _____ Ventricular _____

Conduction: P-R interval _____ QRS duration _____

Configuration/location: P wave _____ QRS complex _____

S-T segment _____ T wave _____

Outstanding features: _____
_____
_____

Diagnosis: _____
_____

Rate: Atrial — *78*   Ventricular — *39*

Rhythm: Atrial — *Regular*   Ventricular — *Regular*

Conduction: P-R — *0.18 sec.*   QRS duration — *0.10 sec.*

Configuration/location: P wave — *Low; precedes QRS.*   QRS complex — *Normal; some absent.*   S-T segment — *Elevated.*   T wave — *Normal.*

Outstanding features: *Atrial rate twice the ventricular rate. Two P waves for every QRS complex. Consistent P-R interval.*

Diagnosis: *Second degree block 2:1*

Rate: Atrial — *65*   Ventricular — *65*

Rhythm: Atrial — *Regular*   Ventricular — *Regular*

Conduction: P-R — *0.20 sec.*   QRS duration — *0.16 sec.*

Configuration/location: P wave — *Tall, peaked; precedes QRS.*   QRS complex — *Wide.*   S-T segment — *Depressed.*   T wave — *Inverted.*

Outstanding features: *Wide QRS complexes with depressed S-T segments and inverted T waves.*

Diagnosis: *Normal sinus rhythm, right bundle branch block*

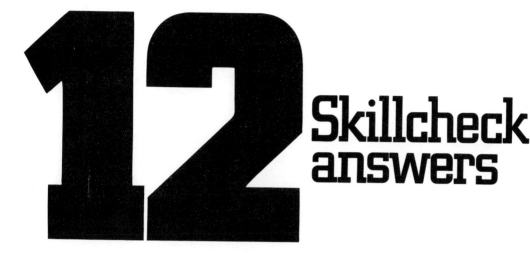

Skillcheck answers

SKILLCHECK 2

1. Atrial and ventricular rates are 60; both rhythms are regular. The P-R interval measures 0.18 seconds, and the QRS duration measures 0.10 seconds. P waves are inverted but precede the QRS complexes. QRS complexes are normal. S-T segments are depressed, and T waves are flattened.

2. Atrial and ventricular rates are 72; both rhythms are regular. The P-R interval measures 0.16 seconds, and the QRS duration measures 0.12 seconds. P waves are normal, preceding the QRS complexes. QRS complexes are slightly widened. S-T segments are elevated, and T waves are peaked.

3. Atrial and ventricular rates are 100; both rhythms are regular. The P-R interval measures 0.20 seconds, and the QRS duration measures 0.10 seconds. P waves are normal, preceding the QRS complexes. QRS complexes are normal, as are S-T segments and T waves.

4. Atrial and ventricular rates are 75; both rhythms are regular. The P-R interval measures 0.20 seconds, and the QRS duration measures 0.10 seconds. The P waves are normal, preceding the QRS complexes. QRS complexes are normal. S-T segments are slightly elevated, and T waves are inverted.

5. Atrial and ventricular rates are 52; both rhythms are regular. The P-R interval measures 0.20 seconds, and the QRS duration measures 0.12 seconds. P waves are flat, but always precede the QRS complexes. QRS complexes are normal, as are the S-T segments. T waves are coved.

SKILLCHECK 3

1. Sinus tachycardia. The clue to this diagnosis is, of course, the rapid atrial and ventricular rates (150). Otherwise, the tracing is normal in every respect (atrial and ventricular rhythms are regular; P-R interval is 0.16 seconds; QRS duration is 0.10 seconds; and configuration and location of all waves is fairly normal).

2. Normal sinus rhythm. This tracing is normal in rate (94), rhythm (regular), conduction (0.17 seconds for the P-R interval, 0.08 seconds for the QRS duration), and configuration of the QRS complex. (P and T waves are slightly rounded and the S-T segments slightly depressed; see chapter 9 for an explanation.)

3. Sinus arrhythmia and bradycardia. Except for the slow atrial and ventricular rates and the slightly irregular atrial and ventricular rhythms, this tracing is normal in rate (53), P-R interval (0.20 seconds), QRS duration (0.10 seconds), and configuration and location of P waves and QRS complexes. (The S-T segment is depressed and T waves are slightly flattened; see chapter 9).

4. Sinus tachycardia. Rates in this tracing are rapid (115). However, the rhythm is regular, the P-R interval is normal (0.18 seconds), and the QRS duration is normal (0.08 seconds). (Notice the slight abnormalities in wave configuration — rounded P waves, coved T waves, and an elevated S-T segment. See chapter 9 for an explanation.)

SKILLCHECK 4

1. Sinus bradycardia with premature atrial contraction. The atrial and ventricular rhythms are slightly irregular, with one short cycle.

2. Atrial fibrillation. The atrial rate is 500. Atrial rhythm is irregular, and ventricular rhythm is grossly irregular. P waves and T waves form an uneven baseline.

3. Atrial fibrillation. The atrial rate is rapid (500). Ventricular rhythm is irregular. P waves and T waves form an uneven baseline.

4. Atrial flutter. Atrial rate is 300. Ventricular rhythm is irregular. P waves and T waves have merged to form sawtooth "F" (flutter) waves.

SKILLCHECK 5

1. Junctional tachycardia. P waves are lost in the QRS complex. QRS complex is normal. Ventricular rate is 72.

2. Junctional rhythm. P waves are either flat or absent, but the QRS is normal. Where measurable, the P-R interval is short. Ventricular rate is 62.

3. Junctional rhythm. P waves are absent, but the QRS is normal. The ventricular rate is 40.

4. Junctional rhythm. P waves are absent, but the QRS is normal. The ventricular rate is 52.

SKILLCHECK 6

1. Normal sinus rhythm with first degree block. The P-R interval is prolonged, at 0.32 seconds.

2. Normal sinus rhythm with first degree block. The P-R interval is prolonged (0.28 seconds).

3. Second degree block, Mobitz II (2:1). The P-R interval is consistent, but the QRS complex is dropped after every other P wave.

4. Second degree block. The P-R interval varies. Ventricular rate varies from 35 to 56, and ventricular rhythm varies with the block (2:1/3:2 conduction).

5. Second degree block, Mobitz II (2:1). The P-R interval is consistent, but the QRS complex is dropped after every other P wave.

SKILLCHECK 7

1. Normal sinus rhythm with premature ventricular contraction. Two QRS complexes deflect in the opposite direction from normal. T waves following the abnormal QRS complexes also deflect in the opposite direction. A compensatory pause follows the abnormal complexes.

2. Asystole. The baseline shows only minimal activity (small waves of excitability appear to come from chest compression).

3. Normal sinus rhythm with premature ventricular contraction. One QRS complex is wide and distorted. The P wave preceding it is flat. There is a compensatory pause after the distorted QRS.

4. Ventricular tachycardia. The QRS complexes are wide and bizarre and occur in rapid succession.

SKILLCHECK 9

1. True infarction of the inferior wall. Leads II, III, and aVF face the inferior surface of the heart. The presence of Q waves and flattened T waves indicates an infarction of the inferior wall of the heart.

2. Muscle injury and ischemia of the anterior wall. Leads I, V_2, and V_3 face the anterior surface of the heart. Slight depression on the S-T segments and inversion of the T waves indicate injury to the anterior myocardium, with resultant ischemia.

3. Current of injury of the inferior wall. Leads II, III, and aVF face the inferior surface of the heart. Elevation of the S-T segments indicates a "current of injury," which indicates possible ischemia of the inferior wall of the heart.

SKILLCHECK 10

1. Muscle tremors.
2. Electrical interference (60-cycle alternating current).
3. Muscle potential (patient movement).

Appendices

TABLE FOR CALIBRATING HEART RATE
(Based on standard of 1500 small EKG squares per minute. *Use for regular rhythm only.*)

NUMBER OF SMALL SQUARES (0.04 sec each)	RATE	NUMBER OF SMALL SQUARES (0.04 sec each)	RATE
3	500	25	60
4	375	26	58
5	300	27	56
6	250	28	54
7	214	29	52
8	188	30	50
9	168	31	48
10	150	32	47
11	136	33	46
12	125	34	44
13	115	35	43
14	107	36	42
15	100	37	41
16	94	38	40
17	88	39	39
18	83	40	38
19	79	41	37
20	75	42	36
21	72	44	35
22	68	46	33
23	65	48	31
24	63	50	30

ATRIAL ARRHYTHMIAS

RHYTHM	MECHANISM AND FEATURES
Normal sinus rhythm	SA node acts as pacemaker. Impulses travel through the normal conduction paths. *EKG features:* Heart rate is 60-100 beats per minute (regular rhythm). P wave precedes each QRS complex. P-R interval is normal.
Sinus bradycardia	Same as normal sinus rhythm except heart rate is below 60 beats per minute.
Sinus tachycardia	Same as normal sinus rhythm except heart rate is over 100 beats per minute but less than 160.
Sinus arrhythmia	SA node acts as pacemaker, but heart rate changes periodically. Heart rate increases with inspiration or decreases with expiration (common in children). *EKG features:* R-R intervals are irregular; P-P intervals vary slightly.
Wandering pacemaker	SA node remains basic pacemaker but heart may also be paced by random foci or AV node. *EKG features:* Ventricular rhythm varies. P waves change configuration or are absent for some beats; P-R interval varies.
Sinus arrest (atrial standstill)	Momentary failure of the SA node to initiate an impulse. Caused by pharyngeal irritation, increased vagal stimulation, anesthesia intubation, carotid sinus massage, or deep inspiration. *EKG features:* Normal sinus rhythm interrupted by an occasional long pause where an entire cardiac cycle (P, QRS, T) is missing. R-R intervals vary because pause isn't equal to two regular cycles.
SA block	Impulse from SA node fails to reach atria; no atrial or ventricular contractions. *EKG features:* Normal sinus rhythm interrupted by an occasional long pause where entire cardiac cycle (P, QRS, T) is missing. Rhythm remains normal because pause is equal to two regular cycles.
Atrial premature contractions (PACs)	An irritable focus in the atria supercedes the SA node as pacemaker for one or more beats. Ventricular conduction is normal. *EKG features:* P waves differ in shape; may be inverted, notched, slurred, flat, or diphasic. P waves also change location, merging with T waves or with QRS complexes.
Atrial tachycardia (PAT)	An irritable focus in the atria increases rate to 160-250 per minute. Onset of PAT is always sudden. *EKG features:* P waves are hidden in QRS, eliminating P-R interval. Rhythm is perfectly regular.

ATRIAL ARRHYTHMIAS

	SIGNIFICANCE	TREATMENT
	Conduction system is operating normally.	None.
	May be normal in athletes but could also indicate atrial disease or myocardial anoxia. Cardiac output is reduced.	If persistent treat with atropine, isoproterenol, or pacemaker.
	Nonspecific; depends on cause (fever, emotional upset, or activity).	Determine and treat cause.
	Innocent disturbance of the normal pacemaker or caused by hyperventilation.	Usually none. Observe patient for other atrial arrhythmias.
	Can occur in normal heart from increased vagal tone. Often found in rheumatic carditis due to tissue inflammation.	Usually none. Determine cause and treat if necessary.
	Important if caused by vagal reactions, e.g., fainting, dizziness, or syncope. Can be caused by digitalis or quinidine excess.	Determine and treat cause. In chronic cases where the patient is symptomatic, insert pacemaker.
	May indicate excess of digitalis or quinidine, vagal stimulation (e.g., carotid massage), or organic heart disease near SA node.	Usually none. Determine cause.
	Dangerous only if more than 6-10 per minute; may develop into paroxysmal atrial tachycardia or atrial fibrillation. Often caused by excess alcohol, tobacco, or food.	If cause is organic, treat disease. Give potassium supplement.
	Serious in organic heart disease. Can cause congestive heart failure.	Give digitalis or quinidine in organic disease. Apply carotid sinus pressure.

ATRIAL ARRHYTHMIAS

RHYTHM	MECHANISM AND FEATURES
Atrial flutter	An irritable focus in the atria takes over pacing. *EKG features:* Atrial rate is 250-350 beats per minute; ventricular rate varies with degree of block in AV conduction. P waves become superimposed on T waves as atrial rate increases, causing a wavy or sawtooth configuration between QRS complexes.
Atrial fibrillation	An atrial ectopic focus discharges more than 400 impulses per minute. Atria lose ability to contract uniformly; atrial walls twitch rather than contract. Only a small percentage of atrial stimuli reaches ventricles. *EKG features:* Ventricular rhythm is irregular. P waves and T waves are replaced by small, irregular, chaotic waves ("f" or fibrillatory waves). QRS complexes are normal in shape and duration (if ventricular block isn't present) but occur irregularly (R-R intervals vary).

ARRHYTHMIAS OF THE AV NODE

RHYTHM	MECHANISM AND FEATURES
Premature junctional contractions (PNCs)	The AV node replaces the SA node as the pacemaker; impulses originate in AV node. Impulse is transmitted to the ventricles and then upward to the atria (retrograde conduction). There are three patterns, depending on origin of impulses. *High (upper node origin)* *EKG features:* P waves occur before QRS complexes; P-R intervals are less than 0.10 seconds. *Mid-nodal* *EKG features:* P waves aren't visible because they are lost in the QRS. *Low nodal* *EKG features:* P waves occur *after* QRS complexes; conduction is retrograde.
Junctional rhythm	Impulses arise in the AV node and control both the ventricles and atria because they spread in both directions. *EKG features:* P waves have the characteristics of PNCs. QRS duration is usually normal. Ventricular rates range from 40 to 60 beats per minute.
Junctional tachycardia	Ventricular rate is 60-200 per minute and may be paroxysmal. *EKG features:* Tracing resembles junctional rhythm except the ventricular rate ranges from 60-100 (slow junctional tachycardia) to 100-220 (rapid junctional tachycardia).

ATRIAL ARRHYTHMIAS

	SIGNIFICANCE	TREATMENT
	Atria aren't contracting normally. May cause congestive failure.	Give digitalis to convert flutter to fibrillation; then give quinidine to treat fibrillation. Other treatments include giving propranolol or DC shock.
	Seen in hyperthyroidism or organic heart disease. Reduces cardiac efficiency by reducing cardiac output. May cause atrial thrombi, increasing risk of embolism.	Give digitalis, quinidine, or propranolol. Other treatment includes DC shock. (Atrial fibrillation is considered under control when ventricular rate is under 100.)

ARRHYTHMIAS OF THE AV NODE

	SIGNIFICANCE	TREATMENT
	Same as PACs.	Usually none. May give potassium or propranolol. Watch for junctional tachycardia
	Can result from excess of digitalis or quinidine. In organic heart disease, rhythm may be permanent.	Give potassium or propranolol.
	Ventricular rates over 150 per minute usually caused by excess of digitalis. Can cause congestive heart failure.	Give potassium, propranolol, small doses of digitalis, or DC shock.

HEART BLOCK

RHYTHM	MECHANISM AND FEATURES
First degree (1⁰) **AV block**	Conduction is normal to the AV node, where impulses are delayed before passing through. *EKG features:* P-R intervals are prolonged to more than 0.21 sec.
Second degree (2⁰) **AV block**	*Wenckebach (Mobitz I):* *EKG features:* P-R intervals vary, becoming progressively longer until a QRS is dropped. Usually there is a cyclic pattern to dropped beats (4:1, 5:1). *Mobitz II* *EKG features:* P-R intervals are fixed, but periodically QRS is dropped. *2:1 AV block* *EKG features:* Every other QRS is dropped.
Third degree (3⁰) **AV block**	Impulses from the atria to the ventricles are blocked, so the atria and ventricles beat independently of each other. There are two pacemakers — one in the atria and one in the ventricles. *EKG features:* Atrial rate is higher than the ventricular rate (ventricular rate is 20-40 beats per minute) and is usually regular. P waves are unrelated to QRS complexes. P-R intervals vary.
AV dissociation	Mechanism is the same as third degree block. There are two pacemakers — one in the atria and the other in the AV node. *EKG features:* Ventricular rate is higher than the atrial rate because ventricles are stimulated from AV node. P waves are unrelated to QRS complexes. P-R intervals vary or are absent.

HEART BLOCK

	SIGNIFICANCE	TREATMENT
	Least dangerous of AV blocks. May be produced by drugs (digitalis and quinidine).	Observe patient for advancing block.
Wenckebach	In 2° block, a narrow QRS means a block in the AV node; a wide QRS means a block in the node-bundle of His system. Dropped beats mean the ventricles aren't contracting rhythmically. Cardiac output is impaired. Ventricular rate is affected by degree of block. 2:1 block is highly dangerous.	Treatment depends on the width of QRS complexes; may require permanent pacing if QRS is wide. Other treatment includes atropine or isoproterenol.
	Causes poor perfusion, Stokes-Adams attacks, PVCs, or ventricular fibrillation.	Doctor must insert a permanent pacemaker.
	Can be caused by digitalis toxicity or disease. Determine cause.	Give atropine to increase the atrial rate by speeding the sinus node. Insert a temporary pacemaker.

VENTRICULAR ARRHYTHMIAS

RHYTHM	MECHANISM AND FEATURES
Bundle branch block	Conduction through the R or L branches of the bundle of His is impaired. Conduction is normal from SA node through the AV node where it is obstructed in one of the branches. The time for complete ventricular stimulation is delayed. *EKG features:* QRS widens to 0.12 sec. or greater.
Premature ventricular contraction (PVC)	Ectopic focus in ventricles stimulates heart before the regularly scheduled SA impulse arrives. *EKG features:* P wave is absent. QRS is wide, bizarre, often going in a different direction from patient's normal QRS. T wave is in opposite direction from QRS.
Ventricular tachycardia	Ventricles are repeatedly stimulated by ectopic foci. This arrhythmia may develop spontaneously but usually occurs with PVCs. *EKG features:* When there are 3 PVCs in a row, ventricular tachycardia exists. P waves may or may not be seen. QRS is wide and bizarre. Rhythm is usually regular.
Ventricular flutter	This arrhythmia appears minutes or seconds before ventricular fibrillation or may follow ventricular tachycardia. *EKG features:* Many multifocal, bizarre PVCs appear. Tracing becomes a wavy, sawtooth configuration with no discernible P, QRS, or T waves.
Ventricular fibrillation	Ventricles are repeatedly stimulated from an ectopic focus so rapidly that the heart can't recover after contractions. *EKG features:* Tracing becomes a series of chaotic waves with no uniformity.
Cardiac arrest (ventricular standstill or asystole)	Electrical force in heart is inadequate to stimulate muscle. Ventricles cease to contract. *EKG features:* Tracing becomes a flat line.

VENTRICULAR ARRHYTHMIAS

	SIGNIFICANCE	TREATMENT
R *L*	May occur in normal patients and cause no symptoms, but underlying damage of upper intraventricular septum is cause for concern.	Usually none. If complicated by advanced AVB, though, insert pacemaker.
	Reflects ventricular irritability. Frequency of occurrence indicates degree of irritability. Dangerous when PVCs are multifocal (coming from more than one foci) or in clusters (2 or more) or when showing R on T pattern.	Give lidocaine bolus and drip, procainamide, quinidine, or diphenylhydantoin (Dilantin).
	Usually denotes myocardial irritability; often precedes ventricular fibrillation. May be transient and self terminating. If sustained will lead to ventricular fibrillation, congestive failure, and cardiogenic shock. May be mistaken for atrial fibrillation or supraventricular tachycardia.	Treatment depends on patient's reaction. If run of ventricular tachycardia is short, give drugs as for PVCs or insert temporary pacemaker. If run is sustained, administer DC shock.
	Dangerous arrhythmia	Administer DC shock.
	Most serious of all arrhythmias. Must treat PVCs and ventricular tachycardia. Must be differentiated from ventricular tachycardia or standstill.	Repeatedly apply DC shock until arrhythmia is reversed. Follow with lidocaine and, if necessary, CPR.
	Transient arrest occurs in Stokes-Adams disease. May be caused by excess digitalis or quinidine, procainamide, or lidocaine, or by straining at defecation.	Give a sharp blow to the chest and administer CPR. Give intracardiac epinephrine. Insert a transthoracic pacemaker.

ANTIARRHYTHMIC AGENTS

GENERIC NAME	TRADE NAME	DOSE
quinidine	Quinidex Quinora Quinaglute Cardioquin	200-300 mg q4-6h, p.o.
procainamide	Pronestyl	250-500 mg q3-6h, p.o.; 0.5-1.0 Gm q4-6h I.M. 1.0-2.0 Gm I.V.
lidocaine	Xylocaine	50-100 mg I.V. bolus, then 1-4 mg/min I.V.
diphenylhydantoin	Dilantin	250-500 mg slow I.V. push, then 200-300 mg q.i.d. or b.i.d.
propranolol	Inderal	1-3 mg I.V. (higher doses have been used); 10-40 mg q.i.d., p.o.

DIGITALIS GLYCOSIDES

GENERIC NAME	TRADE NAME	DIGITALIZATION DOSE	MAINTENANCE DOSE
digitalis leaf (foxglove)	Digifortis Digiglusin Digitora Pil-Digis	1.0-2.0 Gm p.o.	0.05-0.3 Gm p.o.
digitoxin	Crystodigin Digitaline Nativelle Myodigin Purodigin	1.2-2.0 mg p.o.; 1.0-2.0 mg I.V. or I.M.	0.05-0.2 mg p.o.
digoxin	Davoxin Lanoxin	1.0-4.0 mg p.o.; 1.0-2.0 mg I.V. or I.M.	0.25-1.0 mg p.o.
gitalin	Gitaligin	4.0-10.0 mg p.o.	0.25-1.0 mg p.o.
lanatoside C	Cedilanid	5.0-10.0 mg p.o.	0.25-1.0 mg p.o.
deslanoside	Cedilanid-D	1.2-1.0 mg I.V. or I.M.	N.A.
ouabain	G-Strophanthin	0.5-1.0 mg I.V. or I.M.	N.A.
acetyldigitoxin	Acylanid	1.6-2.2 mg p.o.	0.1-0.2 mg p.o.

ANTIARRHYTHMIC AGENTS

ADVERSE EFFECTS	EKG CHANGES
cichonism (nausea and vomiting, diarrhea, tinnitus, salivation, vertigo, visual disturbances), thrombocytopenia, rash, hypotension	*Normal:* prolonged QRS *Abnormal:* 2⁰ or complete block, PVCs, ventricular arrhythmias
GI and CNS disturbances, hypotension, bone marrow depression, agranulocytosis, fever, allergic reactions, systemic lupus-like syndrome (positive LE prep)	*Normal:* widened QRS complex *Abnormal:* tachycardia
drowsiness (often desirable effect), CNS disturbances, convulsions (give diazepam, 10 mg I.V.), hypotension	*Abnormal:* heart block
hypotension, CNS disturbances, rash, hypoplasia of gums	*Abnormal:* heart block, bradycardia
heart failure, hypotension, bronchoconstriction, GI and CNS disturbances, rash, paresthesias, hypoglycemia	*Normal:* prolonged P-R interval *Abnormal:* heart block

DIGITALIS GLYCOSIDES

ADVERSE EFFECTS	EKG CHANGES
anorexia, nausea, vomiting and diarrhea, lethargy, drowsiness, confusion, visual changes	
mental depression, anorexia, nausea, vomiting, restlessness, yellow vision, mental confusion, disorientation, delirium	
anorexia, nausea, vomiting.	*Normal:* prolonged P-R interval *Abnormal:* PACs, PVCs, ventricular and supraventricular tachycardias, heart block, AV dissociation, junctional rhythm
anorexia, nausea, vomiting, diarrhea, headache, weakness, apathy, visual disturbances	
anorexia, nausea and vomiting, blurred vision, flickering objects of green and yellow, disorientation	
anorexia, nausea, vomiting, diarrhea, headache, weakness, apathy, visual disturbances	
anorexia, nausea and vomiting, blurred vision, flickering objects of green and yellow, disorientation	
anorexia, nausea, vomiting, diarrhea, headache, weakness, apathy, visual disturbances	

GLOSSARY

anoxia: A deficiency of oxygen in body tissues, due to reduction in blood flow or other causes.

arrhythmia: Any disturbance in the normal rhythm of the heart beat; irregularities may occur in discharge of impulses from the SA node or in conduction of impulses through heart tissue.

atherosclerosis: A common form of arteriosclerosis in which deposits of yellow, fatty plaques build up in the arteries; may cause arterial occlusion.

bigeminy: Any condition that occurs in pairs, particularly two beats of the pulse in rapid succession followed by a pause.

bradycardia: An abnormally slow heart rate.

cardiac output: Amount of blood discharged by either ventricle per minute.

cardioversion: Conversion of an arrhythmia to normal sinus rhythm by electrical shocks.

carotid sinus: A dilated portion of the common carotid artery, just above the bifurcation of the two main branches, containing a rich supply of nerve endings from the sinus branch of the vagus nerve.

carotid sinus pressure (or massage): Manual pressure applied on the carotid sinus; this slows the heart rate.

circus movement: The theory that an electrical impulse originates in one area, travels in a circular path, and re-enters in the same area to produce a cycle (a possible mechanism for atrial flutter and fibrillation).

congestive heart failure: Failure of the heart to maintain adequate blood circulation, causing breathlessness, weakness, and abnormal sodium and water retention. This condition is caused by heart disease and may cause congestion in the lungs or in peripheral circulation.

coronary visualization (cardiac angiography): X-ray examination of the coronary arteries after a radiopaque dye has been injected into them.

ECG: see EKG

ectopic focus: A focus other than the normal one. In cardiology, a source of cardiac stimulus other than the SA node, usually caused by some irritation of the myocardium.

EKG or ECG: Electrocardiogram; a graphic tracing of electrical activity of the heart.

electrocardiogram: see EKG

electrocardiograph: An instrument for making electrocardiograms.

extrasystole: A contraction of the heart that occurs prematurely and interrupts the normal rhythm.

fibrillation: Quivering or uncoordinated muscle contraction.

heart block: Impairment of cardiac conduction so that electrical impulses from the atria fail to pass through the AV node to the ventricles.

hypoxia: Low oxygen content.

infarct: Localized tissue death caused by ischemia to the area. Myocardial infarction refers to an infarct of the heart muscle.

ischemia: Localized deficiency of blood caused by constriction or obstruction of the blood vessel to the area.

MI: Myocardial infarction; infarct of the myocardium, usually resulting from myocardial ischemia following occlusion of a coronary artery.

mitral stenosis: Stricture or narrowing of the mitral valve or orifice; usually caused by rheumatic fever.

pacemaker: The SA node, so called because it initiates the electrical impulses that set the rhythm of cardiac contractions. An *artificial pacemaker* is an electrical device to pace cardiac rhythm, used particularly when a patient has heart block.

parasystole: An arrhythmia caused by two foci, usually the SA node and an ectopic focus in the ventricle, independently initiating cardiac impulses.

paroxysmal: Recurring suddenly and abruptly.

rule of bigeminy: The theory that PVCs tend to occur with low heart rates.

Stokes-Adams syndrome: Sudden attacks of unconsciousness, sometimes coupled with convulsions, which may accompany heart block or ventricular arrythmia both producing low cardiac outputs.

systole: Contraction of the heart, which causes ejection of blood from the heart chambers into the circulatory system.

tachycardia: An abnormally fast heart rate.

vagus nerve: The tenth cranial nerve, part of the parasympathetic nervous system. When stimulated, the vagus nerve slows the heart rate.

vagal stimulation: Pharmacologic or manual stimulation of the vagus nerve to slow the heart rate.

Valsalva's maneuver: Bearing down, or forced exhalation effort against a closed glottis, which slows the heart rate.

FOR FURTHER REFERENCE

Dubin, Dale. *Rapid Interpretation of EKGs, 2nd Edition.* New York: Cover Publishing Co., 1972. (This programmed text seems to be a favorite of beginners.)

Friedberg, Charles K. *Diseases of the Heart, Third Edition.* Philadelphia: W.B. Saunders Company, 1966.

Goldman, Mervin. *Principles of Clinical Electrocardiography.* Los Altos, Calif.: Lange Medical Publications, 1970.

Ownby, Fred, ed. *Advanced Cardiac Nursing.* Philadelphia: The Charles Press, 1970. (Good for continuing education.)

Sharp, LaVaughn and Beatrice Rabin. *Nursing in the Coronary Care Unit.* Philadelphia: J.B. Lippincott Co., 1970. (This reference book includes the clinical symptoms associated with each arrhythmia.)

Index